From The Shepherd's Purse

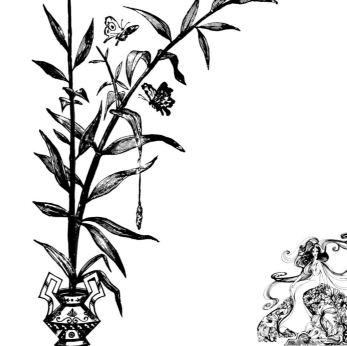

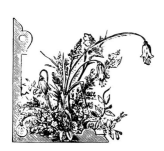

CREDITS

ILLUSTRATORS

Dave Story - Kennewick, Washington

S. D. Lowder - Pocatello, Idaho

M. G. Barlow - McCammon, Idaho

PLANT PHOTOGRAPHERS

Robert Jensen - Pocatello, Idaho

S. L. Welsh - Provo, Utah

Lloyd Beesley - Cedar Grove, Indiana

Chuck Andrews - Naha, Okinawa

R. M. Housenecht - Monroeton, Penn.

Bill Ratcliff - Orem, Utah

W. S. Justice - Asheville, N. Carolina

M. G. Barlow - McCammon, Idaho

COVER

Media Synthesis - Ojai, California

TYPESETTING

Litho Printing - Pocatello, Idaho

LAYOUTS

Lowder Art & Ad Service - Pocatello, Idaho

From The Shepherd's Purse

The Identification, Preparation and Use
of Medicinal Plants

BY MAX G. BARLOW

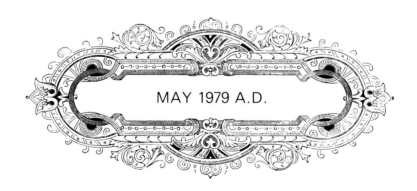

MAY 1979 A.D.

Library of Congress
Catalog Card No.   79-65086

ISBN   0-9602812-0-7

FOREWORD

There is a great need for a good botanical work on medicinal plants. This need has been satisfied with the publication of this book. I have watched the development and formation of this scholarly work from its inception nearly ten years ago. The author's keen interest in botanicals, combined with his scientific training and research, makes this one of the best texts available for anyone genuinely interested in obtaining a good working knowledge of medicinal plants, their identification, preparation and use.

This book is written for those desiring to learn which plants may be of service to them in case of an emergency, or to merely strengthen their knowledge of a once very useful art.

As you can quickly observe, much work has gone into making this a practical book. The charts and color-coding will save much time and guess-work when collecting plants and preparing them for use.

Max Barlow's skill as a botanist combined with his talent as a writer, makes this book a unique contribution to the field of herbology. He has done extensive research into the medicinal uses of botanicals, and has a rich background in the medicinal-nutritional field. He is presently working with Dr. E.T. Krebs, Jr. on several important projects, one being a very effective natural plant respiratory antibiotic.

Next in line for publication will be his book on poisonous and edible plants.

Dr. Milton P. Nelson, N.D.

FROM THE SHEPHERD'S PURSE
TABLE OF CONTENTS

DEDICATION

To my Dad and Mother for their sustaining influence in
my life, and for their helping me to love freedom and
liberty.

ACKNOWLEDGEMENTS

I wish to express my love for Dr. and Mary Nelson for their constant support and encouragement. It is an honor to be their friend.

To S. D. Lowder, for his excellent work in the technical construction of this book. Also to Litho Printing for their fine typesetting.

Paragon Press was most helpful in seeing that only the best of workmanship and materials went into the construction of this book.

To Dr. Bill Eakin, owner of Bridgeport Press, for his timely assistance and for his efforts in marketing and distribution of this work.

Special thanks to my illustrators and photographers for their expertise.

To Dr. Stan Welsh and Dr. Joseph Murdock of Brigham Young University, who, many years ago inspired me to work with plants; and for the many enjoyable hours in the field where I received excellent instruction in Plant Taxonomy.

To my Brother and Sister - for their faith in me.

To my four boys and eight girls who went without their father so that this book could be.

To my good friends - Dr. E. T. Krebs, Jr., and Miss Malvina Cassese for their help.

To my good wife Anne, who knew this project could be completed and who encouraged me every step of the way. Without her help, this book would have been next to impossible to complete.

Finally, to *Him* who causes the Flower to grow.

PREFACE

Today more and more people are becoming interested in the Natural Healing Arts. There is a general feeling among people today to know how to be self-sufficient and to care for ones own general welfare. Established institutions seem to be becoming less and less able to provide the security that many wish to maintain or to acquire.

Collecting and using natural herbs is a serious business and should be done with soberness and with good judgement. Many people are poisoned each year in the attempt to use plants for medicinal purposes. Fortunately, not many are fatal.

This book is written to aid those interested in collecting and using botanicals for healing purposes. Full color pictures of the plants are included because proper identificatin is vital where there is a possibility of using the wrong plant.

I made a complete review of practically all that has been written on the subject and came to the conclusion that something was lacking. Simply listing a plant and what it was reported to do left most people wondering, where do I find this plant? And once I locate it, what then? Many serious errors were also made in the classification of the plants.

Reputed ''cures'' varied from book to book. Medicinal uses listed in this book were checked with reliable contemporary practitioners and cross-referenced with some of the practitioners of the past. I have used many of the plants included in this book and know the great benefit they offer. Official Pharmacopoeias and Formularies (Both American and British) were also used to verify the healing status of the plant.

Most of the plants listed in this book are extremely safe to use, but care must still be exercised because body chemistries differ and where a reaction occurs, immediately discontinued use is the responsible action.

This book is written to assist you in maintaining proper physical health. Proper functioning of the body is dependent upon many factors. The relationship of body and mind must be kept in healthy balance. Proper diet, honest hard work, daily exercise, stimulating intellectual development and positive social interactions with good people will greatly assist in proper maintenance of body physiology.

Nutrition based primarily with foods which, in the past, have been part of the "biological experience" should make up the bulk of your diet. Millet, whole wheat, fresh fruits and vegetables (eaten with as little cooking as possible) should be the center of your food intake. Stay away from processed foods as much as possible.

Food supplementation is necessary, but should be wisely selected and put into its proper perspective. Proper eating of wholesome foods should always preceed supplementation.

When selecting plants for medicinal uses, only those of healthy specimens should be collected. Sanitary conditions and preparation techniques are vitally important to the success of your work with herbs. Collect plants away from chemical sprays or where roadside pollutants have contaminated the area.

Care should be taken not to damage existing plant populations which are rare or in danger of extinction. Many of the plants listed in this book can be cultivated and should be for the preservation of some of our wild flowers. Property rights of those where the plant might be found growing, should be honored completely.

It will be observed that when preparing some of the plants for use as described in the preparations section, other ways more suitable to your situation may be better. I recommend that you experiment with various techniques which will give you better results. You will find that preparation is an art which must be developed.

Tinctures and Fluid Extracts calling for alcohol preparations should use only ethyl alcohol or grain alcohol. **Denatured or wood alcohols must not be used for they are toxic and poisonous.** Care must also be taken not to have an open flame near alcohol for it is very flammable and can cause serious burns to the skin.

Ointments will be fun to work with. You will be surprised with some of "your creations". You will have to adjust your ointment preparations with the climatic conditions in your area. Temperature will be the main consideration.

Infusion and Decoctions are extracting methods which use water. The main thing to remember with these extracting techniques is that they are only temporary preparations, and the unused portions will need to be discarded several hours after preparation.

Powdering plants will take special equipment which will be discussed in the Powdering Preparation section. A source of supply will be listed to aid you in acquiring powdering equipment at the end of this preface.

Two very important sections are included in this book. Plant Morphology and Plant Taxonomy. Morphology deals with studying plant structures which are used to identify plants. Taxonomy is another term for a process of plant identification. A very simple yet easy method showing the process of identification by way of elimination is included to teach the methods used by botanists to identify a plant.

The weight and measure information is found on pages 177-178 and will help you formulate the proper amounts of dried herbs used in each plant preparation. The amount of herbs used and the amount of extracting solvent is given in the English measurements of ounces and pints or quarts. Dosages of Tinctures, Powders, and Fluid Extracts are given in the Apothecary with metric equivalents. (see chart p. 178)

Dosages should be calculated and regulated for children, women, and the aged. The dosages recommended in this book is for a man of approximately 150 pounds.

In calculating the child's dosage, one of the following rules may be followed:

CLARK'S RULE:

$$\frac{\text{Weight of child in pounds}}{\text{150 Pounds (Ave. adult wt.)}} = \text{Fraction of adult dose to be used}$$

COWLING'S RULE:

$$\frac{\text{Child's age (on next bithday)}}{24} = \text{Fraction of adult dose to be used}$$

YOUNG'S RULE:

$$\frac{\text{Child's age } + \text{ 12 years}}{\text{Child's age}} = \text{Fraction of adult dose to be used}$$

Young's Rule is the one most frequently used, but for more scientific accuracy, Clark's Rule should be followed because it recognizes the application of the therapeutic agent to the body's surface which is particularily applicable to women who, as a general rule, require smaller doses than men.

To assist those wishing to obtain quality materials necessary for making medicinal plant preparation, the Royal Botanical Company has all the available equipment (powdering and extracting equipment) and materials (ointment bases, extracting solvents*, etc.) necessary for your basic preparation of Botanicals. Most of the equipment referred to throughout this book can be obtained from R.B.C. Other medicinal plants not listed in the text of this book are available in monographic form. For a complete catalog of materials, equipments, plant monographs, and other Botanical information -Send $1.00 and a stamped self-addressed (legal size) envelope to:

ROYAL BOTANICAL COMPANY
P.O. BOX 2054
POCATELLO, IDAHO 83201

*Alcohol (ethyl) is not available from R.B.C., but can be purchased commercially at retail outlets. CAUTION: Do not use wood alcohol, rubbing alcohol, or alcohol labeled denatured.

HOW TO USE THE BOOK

PLANT PARTS USED: This collecting data is put in convenient chart form to assist those desiring to collect botanicals for medicinal purposes. Not all plant parts contain medicinal properties. Some plant structures totally lack healing agents, while other plant parts may be harmful to use. This is not always the case, but in some instances it holds true. In some plants, only the flowers are to be used (Arnica), in others, only the roots are used (Leptotaenia). The roots of the Elderberry should never be used (Poison). Root collecting is generally done in the Spring or late Summer when the plant medicines are concentrated below the surface of the ground. Spring collections require pre-marking to locate the roots. Annual plants (those requiring only one growing season to complete their life cycle) generally do not develop massive root systems and can be used with the other plant parts used.

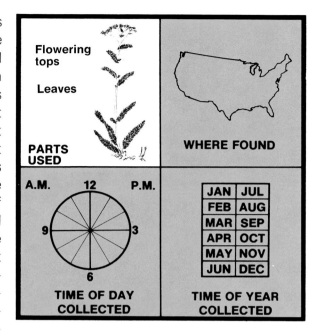

TIME OF DAY COLLECTED: Three factors need to be kept in mind concerning the collecting time. **One** — Plants should be collected after the morning dew and other moisture has evaporated. This is to prevent mildew and rotting of plants you plan to store for later use. **Two** — In some plants the active principle is at its highest potency when the plant's photosynethetic machinery is going at its full capacity. (This is normally when the sun is at its zenith relative to the plant position, approximately between the hours of 11 a.m. and 2 p.m.) Most plant chemicals remain stable once they are formed, while others become essentially worthless during the plant's ''resting'' time. This is especially true of the plants containing glucosides. **Three** — The last factor is self-evident. Plants should be collected when there is enough light to properly identify the plant and discard diseased or inferior plant parts.

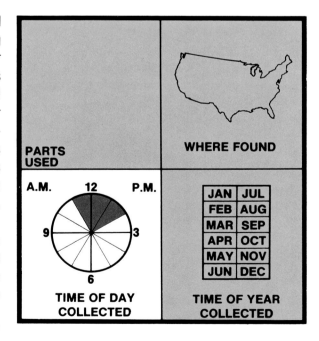

WHERE FOUND. Many of the plants in this book are found world-wide. Many can and should be cultivated. (Cultivated plants are so designated). Plants and plant communities are not static but dynamic and are subject to the constant environmental pressures and condition changes and to the influences of man's activities. Therefore, in many cases, the exact geographical locality of a plant cannot be marked. For example, Blessed Thistle, a plant thought to be a more southeastern plant, has now been found as far west and north as central Utah. Many of the plants are constant companions of man and can be found co-habitating with him. Probably nine or ten plants, listed as medicinal in this book, can be found within 100 feet of your home. Careful observation will help you become familiar with many useful nearby plants.

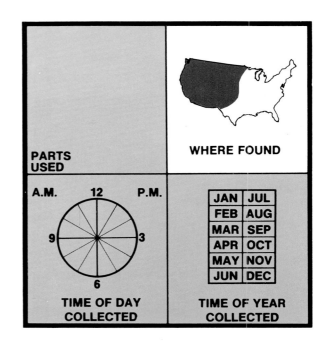

When you are on a field trip, a note pad is helpful for making notes on localities of medicinal and edible plants you have discovered. This information may be recorded later in the margins next to the picture of the plant.

TIME OF YEAR COLLECTED. Plants are most often ready for collection just as the flower is about to open for the first time. (anthesis). This time will vary greatly depending upon climatic conditions, seasonal fluctuations, elevation, North and South Latitudes, etc. The higher the elevation and the more northerly a plant grows, the later in the spring or summer the plant can be collected. Conversely, the lower the elevation and the farther south a plant is found growing, the sooner its flowering time arrives and the sooner it can be collected. Root collection is normally restricted to the late summer or to the early spring. When possible, collections should take place when conditions for drying and storage will be ideal.

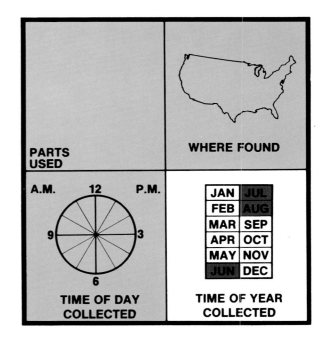

COLOR CODING

The Medicinal Use Section and the Preparation Section (found opposite each other) is designed to help match the ailment with the suggested preparation techniques for the ailment. Match the Medicinal Use Color with the same Preparation color given on the adjoining page.

Each different type of preparation lists a Section number for those needing additional information in the proper preparation of plant medicines. These sections give basic information for each type of preparation considered. This is to broaden your understanding of plant preparation techniques. For example, when preparing an ointment, it is suggested you refer to Section 5 (pages 88 and 89) to review important information regarding the general preparation of ointment.

Proper diagnosis by a qualified physician is a must before a person starts to administer medicinal herbs. Improper use could bring serious results if the actual cause of the illness is different from the manifested form of the sickness. These Preparation Sections are in no way designed for diagnostic procedures or considerations.

MEDICINAL USES:

- Fever
- Colic
- Flatulence

Produces Urination where it has stopped.

PREPARATION:

Infusion (See Section 7 for General Infusion Preparation Information)

STANDARD INFUSION

Dosage: Adult 2 tablespoonsful Q.I.D.

PLANT NAMES

Both the common and botanical names are listed. Most people become confused and fearful when they hear "Scientific Names" attached to a plant, claiming they are "too big" and too difficult to spell and pronounce. To a large extent this is true, however, using both genus and species names are vitally important when trying to correctly identify a plant.

Also much can be learned from the common and scientific names. For example, consider plant #35, the common dandelion. The name comes from the French, *dent de lion,* so named because the leaf margins resemble the "teeth of the Lion".

The genus name *Taraxacum* and the species name *officinale* have important meanings. The Greek word *tarassein,* means "to stir up", and *officinale* refers to the plant being an official medicinal plant of the ancient Roman and Greek governments.

Common names change from place to place. The Plant called Red Root by some people is called Pig Weed by others. They lack standardization and oftimes lead to confusion.

Scientific or Botanical names remain constant. The plant *Amaranthus retroflexus* (Red Root or Pig Weed) is called the same no matter in which country it is found growing. All Scientists use the Latin terminology to avoid errors in plant identification.

All of the plants given scientific names in this book are considered medicinal. This is not true of all plant species in a genus. For example, Pleurisy Root, *Asclepias tuberosa,* is a useful medicinal plant, but *Asclepias speciosis* the common milk weed has no healing properties, but is an edible plant.

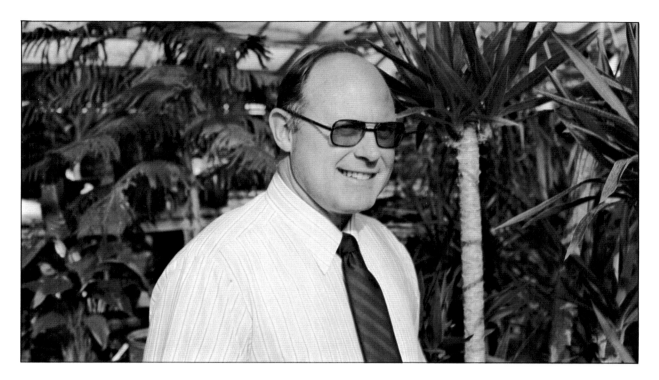

The author is a native of Utah. He was educated in Oregon, Idaho and in Utah where he received his degree from the Brigham Young University. His undergraduate work centered in Botany and Zoology with special emphasis in Pre-medicine, Medical Arthropodology, Endocrinology, Human Physiology and Anatomy. His graduate program focused primarily on Plant Taxonomy.

He has spent hours in the field conducting plant research. He served as a Range Research Technician for the U.S. Forest Service in the mountains of Idaho and was priviledged to work with the outstanding botanist, Ralph Holmgren, at the Desert Experimental Range in the West Utah desert.

Because of his expertise in the field of useful plants (medicinal and edible) he is oftimes asked to serve as Ranger Botanist on Desert Survival expeditions. He has spent many hours doing field research and is considered a Western authority of medicinal plants.

This past year he has been working with Dr. E. T. Krebs, Jr., of San Francisco, on the medicinal plant *Leptotaenia dissecta* studying its antibiotic-antiviral effects on the pulmonary and urinary systems. He is planning a doctorate program and plans to continue his studies in plant medicines.

Max and his Wife, Anne Marie and family, reside in Southeastern Idaho.

The Publishers

Section I

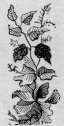

Shepherd's Purse

The Internal Bleeding Healer

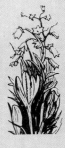

Comfrey

The Bone Mender

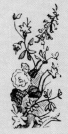

Mullein

The Lung and Wind-pipe Healer

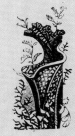

Garlic

The "Bad" Germ Fighter

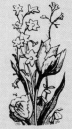

Red Clover

The Blood Purifier

PLANT IDENTIFICATION #1

SHEPHERD'S PURSE

Lady's Purse, Mother's Heart
Case Weed, Blind Weed
Shepherd's Bag, Shepherd's Sprouts
Witches Pouches, Rattle Pouches

CAPSELLA BURSA-PASTORIS

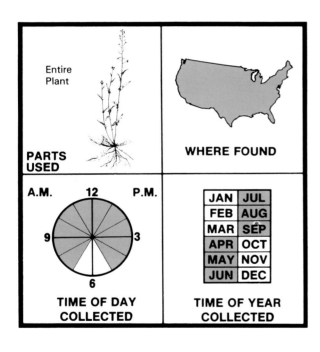

Entire Plant

PARTS USED

WHERE FOUND

A.M.   12   P.M.

9   3

6

TIME OF DAY COLLECTED

JAN	JUL
FEB	AUG
MAR	SEP
APR	OCT
MAY	NOV
JUN	DEC

TIME OF YEAR COLLECTED

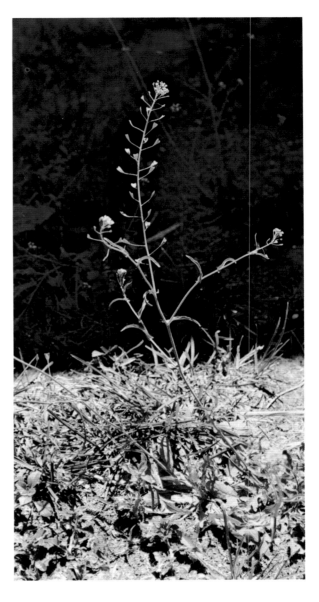

MEDICINAL USES:

- All types of internal hemorrhages:
- After childbirth
- Bloody urine
- Bleeding from the the lungs
- Bleeding stomach
- Profuse menstruation
- Dropsy
- Nosebleeds

- Nose bleeds
- Cuts
- Wounds
- Earache

- Wounds (especially of the head)

- Nose bleeds
- Cuts
- Wounds
- Earache

PLANT INFORMATION:

Shepherd's Purse belongs to the Mustard Family (Cruciferae). It is so named because the ripened seed pod resembles an old-fashioned leather Shepherd's Purse. (See cover of book)

The whole plant is to be used.

It is to be used just prior to, or immediately after parturition (child birth) to prevent or to stop hemorrhaging.

Capsella is rich in Vitamins C and K.

It is a lawn weed and can be found along roadsides and in moist areas around living quarters. Weather permitting, it will grow the year around.

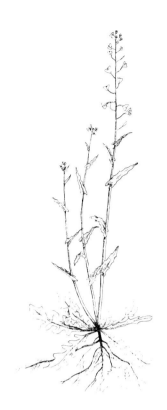

PREPARATION:

INFUSION (See Section 7 for General Infusion Preparation Information)

Pour 12 oz. boiling water over 1 oz. fresh green plant. Steep for 30 minutes. Cool and drink.

Dosage: Wineglassful Q.I.D.

Note: Use ½ oz. if dried plant is used.

OINTMENT (See Section 5 for General Ointment Preparation Information)

Use 8 oz. fresh plant and 16 oz. lard. Contuse the plant to a pulp and add to melted lard. Heat over direct flame until moisture evaporates. Strain through clean cloth and place in jar for later use.

POULTICE (See Section 4 for General Poultice Preparation Information)

Crush and bruise leaves, moisten with hot water. Cover with a sterile cloth to keep moist and in place.

EMERGENCY/Field Use

For earache: Crush plant to a pulp. Squeeze several drops into ear. Place cotton at ear opening. For Nose Bleed: Pound or chew plant into a moist pulp and insert into bleeding nostril(s).

MEDICINAL PROPERTIES

Hemostatic
Mild Astringent
Diuretic
Antihemorrhagic
Mild Stimulant

PLANT IDENTIFICATION #2

COMFREY

Knitbone, Healing Herb
Wallwort, Black Root
Knitback, Gum Plant
Consound, Bruisewort

SYMPHYTUM OFFICINALE

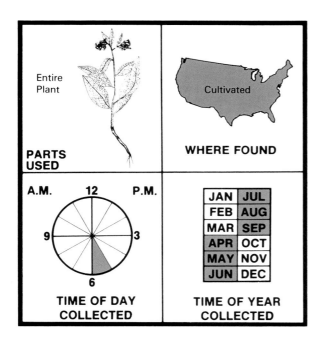

Entire Plant	Cultivated
PARTS USED	**WHERE FOUND**
A.M. 12 P.M. / 9 — 3 / 6	JAN JUL / FEB AUG / MAR SEP / APR OCT / MAY NOV / JUN DEC
TIME OF DAY COLLECTED	**TIME OF YEAR COLLECTED**

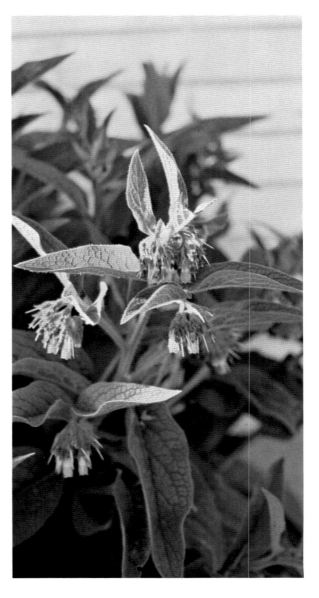

MEDICINAL USES:

- Diarrhea
- Dysentery
- Coughs
- Bleeding lungs
- Internal pains & bruises
- Leukorrhea (as a douche)
- Broken or crushed bones (Light green leaves)

- Diarrhea
- Dysentery
- Coughs
- Bleeding lungs
- Internal pains & bruises
- Leukorrhea (as a douche)
- Broken or crushed Bones

- Ulcerous and odoriferous sores
- Traumatic injury to the eye
- Broken and crushed bones
- Amputations
- Burns

- Diarrhea
- Dysentery
- Coughs
- Bleeding lungs
- Internal pains and bruises
- Leukorrhea (as a douche)
- Broken or crushed bones

PLANT INFORMATION:

Symphytum is in the Borage Family (Boraginaceae).

Comfrey is an excellent plant to cultivate for year around use. It grows best in a shady environment and reproduces by seed or by vegetative division of the roots in the fall. The roots are very brittle and only a small part will grow into a new plant.

The name Comfrey indicates one of its therapeutic uses, *con firma* referring to the uniting of bones.

The botanical name Symphytum is derived from the Greek word *sympho,* to unite.

Its use as a vulnerary is due to its ability to reduce swelling in the fractured area, allowing the union of the bones to take place.

It is rich in vitamins and minerals. It contains vitamins B_1, Pantothenic Acid, B_2, C, B_{12}, E, Allantoin, Iron, Manganese, Calcium, Phosphorus.

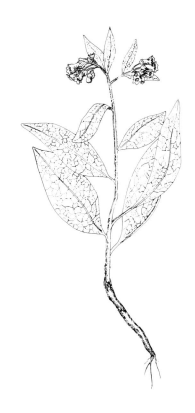

PREPARATION:

INFUSION (See Section 7 for General Infusion Preparation Information)

Prepare leaves and stem in standard infusion, steep 20 minutes, cool and strain.

Dosage: Take frequently in wineglassful amounts every 2 or 3 hours.

DECOCTION (See Section 7 for General Decoction Preparation Information)

Prepare as for standard decoction, boil for 20 min. in water or milk. Cool and strain.

Dosage: Take frequently in wineglassful amounts every 2 or 3 hours.

POULTICE (See Section 4 for General Poultice Preparation Information)

Chop leaves and stem in blender. Add hot water to warm poultice. Squeeze out excess moisture. Cover with moist cloth and a piece of plastic to prevent clothing from being stained by the plants chlorophyll.

Powdered root: moisten into a paste and apply as above.

FLUID EXTRACT (See Section 6 for General Fluid Extract Preparation Information)

Prepare as — STANDARD FLUID EXTRACT

Dosage: ½ to 2 drachms in warm water Q.I.D.

MEDICINAL PROPERTIES

Demulcent
Vulnerary
Pectoral
Astringent

Excellent Substitute of Coffee

COMBINATIONS

Equal parts of
dried Comfrey Root
Dried Dandelion
Root and
Dried
Chicory
(No harmful side effects)

Infusion

PLANT IDENTIFICATION #3

MULLEIN
Torches, Mullein Dock
Blanket Herb, Rag Paper
Candle Wick Plant, Jacobs Staff
Wild Ice, Shepherds Staff
Adams Flannel, Felt Wart
Old Man's Flannel

VERBASCUM THAPSUS

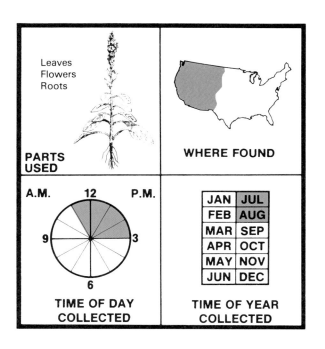

Leaves
Flowers
Roots

PARTS USED

WHERE FOUND

A.M. 12 P.M.
9 3
6

TIME OF DAY COLLECTED

JAN	JUL
FEB	AUG
MAR	SEP
APR	OCT
MAY	NOV
JUN	DEC

TIME OF YEAR COLLECTED

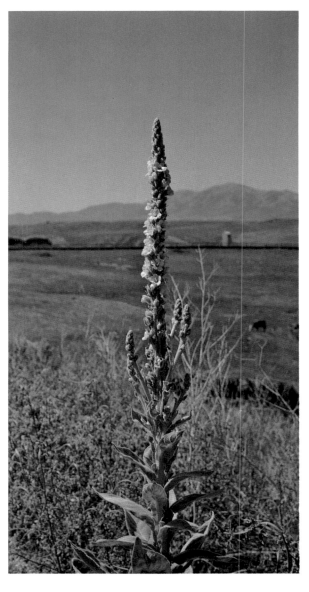

MEDICINAL USES:

- Dysuria
- Cystitis
- Amenorrhea
- Mastitis (Fomentation)
- Bronchitis
- Asthma

- Dysuria
- Cystitis
- Amenorrhea
- Bactericide

- Ringworm
- Bactericide

- Earache
- Mumps
- Bactericide

PLANT INFORMATION:

Mullein is in the Snapdragon Family (Scrophulariaceae) and has many medicinal uses. This plant is a biennial requiring two growing seasons to complete its life cycle.

The name Verbascum (Latin) is thought to be a corruption of the word barbascum, meaning beard, referring to the shaggy pubescence of its leaves and stems.

The seeds have been used to catch fish. The seeds are narcotic and when thrown in very slow moving water will cause temporary stupor in fish.

The dry leaves make excellent tinder and will readily ignite with the slightest spark making it an excellent emergency fire starting plant. Mullein and dried thistle heads make the best emergency starting material available in the out-of-doors.

The leaves cut into long strips and dried have been used as oil lamp wicks.

Some asthmatics have obtained relief by rolling the dried leaves and smoking them.

It is easy to locate this plant because the elongated stem is persistant for about one year after it dies.

The plant is rich in iron, magnesium, potassium, sulfur and calcium phosphate.

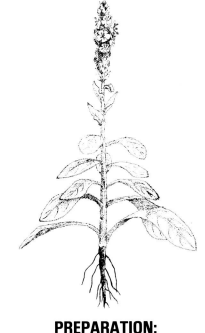

PREPARATION:

DECOCTION (See Section 7 for General Decoction Preparation Information)

STANDARD DECOCTION

Dosage: 1 tablespoonful T.I.D. or Q.I.D.

POWDER (See Section 8 for General Powder Preparation Information)

Grind dried plant into a powder, mix with honey to make a paste. Apply to infected area.

OIL OF MULLEIN
(Special Preparation)

(1) Remove the flowers from stem, place in small container of Olive Oil. Soak (Macerate) for 3 weeks in warm sunlight, or near a warm stove.

(2) Remove the flowers from the stem. Place in tightly corked clear glass jar. Hang bottle in sun for 4 weeks. Oil from flower will have been distilled. Add 10% alcohol - mix.

Place 2 or 3 drops in aching or purulent ear.

INFUSION (See Section 7 for General Infusion Preparation Information)

STANDARD INFUSION

Dosage: 1 wineglassful T.I.D. or Q.I.D.

MEDICINAL PROPERTIES

Demulcent, Emollient
Astringent, Anodyne (Pectoral)
Slightly dedative and narcotic

COMBINATIONS

Bronchitis & Asthma 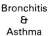 Equal Parts Mullein Lobelia — Standard Infusion

PLANT IDENTIFICATION #4

GARLIC
Garlic

ALLIUM SATIVUM
Allium campanulatum
Allium species

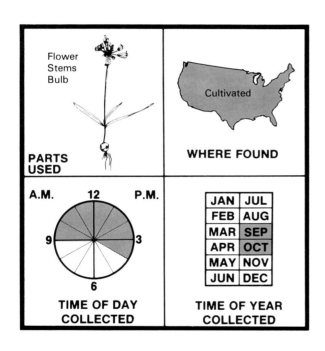

Flower Stems Bulb **PARTS USED**	Cultivated **WHERE FOUND**
A.M. 12 P.M. 9 · 3 6 **TIME OF DAY COLLECTED**	JAN JUL FEB AUG MAR SEP APR OCT MAY NOV JUN DEC **TIME OF YEAR COLLECTED**

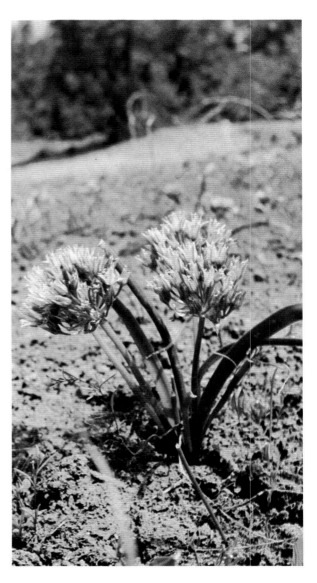

MEDICINAL USES:

- Infections
- Suppuration

- Rheumatic Pains

A

- Asthma
- Whooping Cough
- Bronchitis

B

- Asthma
- Coughs
- Bronchitis
- Strep Throat

C

PLANT INFORMATION:

Garlic is in the Lily Family (Liliaceae). It was used extensively as the primary infection fighter during WW I. (before the availability of the sulfa drugs and penicillin) to combat suppuration resulting from battle wounds. It is still an excellent bacteriocide, destroying pathogenic bacteria while leaving the beneficial ones unharmed.

This plant may be collected from the ground at most any time of the year. The best time to collect the bulbs is about one week after the first fall frost (as indicated by the dead stems and leaves).

Use a little personal creativity when you prepare garlic for medicinal treatments. Do not use aluminum cookware. Use stainless steel, corning ware, porcelain, or heat resistant glass ware, when preparing this plant.

Wild garlic and wild onion leaves and stems can be mashed and bruised by vigorously rubbing them between your hands and applying the expressed juices to the exposed skin to ward off insects.

Garlic is an excellent source of organic sulphur. More people should learn to accept the aroma rather than consider it an objectionable odor.

OINTMENT (See Section 5 for General Ointment Preparation Instructions)
Express juice from 3 to 4 bulbs. Mix juice with less than 1 lb. of lard. Rub on chest and throat as needed. Or mix with vaseline (less than 1 lb.) rub on bottom of the feet.

MEDICINAL PROPERTIES
Antiseptic, Antispasmodic
Diaphoretic, Diuretic, Expectorant

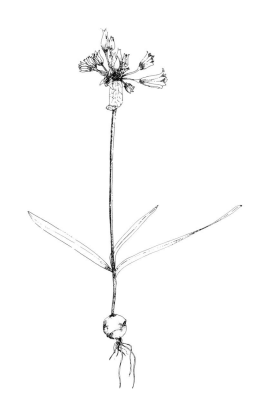

PREPARATION:

OIL OF GARLIC (Special Preparation)
Grate and bruise garlic cloves, place to a depth of 1″ in ½ qt. container or jar. Cover with fresh, pure olive oil. Place in sun or warm place for 3 full days. Strain and bottle, store in cool place.

Dosage: Use as needed.

A

PLANT JUICE (Special Preparation)
Mix 1 part expressed juice with 2 parts distilled water. Apply mixture with cotton swab to infected sore or wound.

B

SYRUP OF GARLIC (Special Preparation)
Pour 1 qt. of boiling water on 1 lb. of sliced garlic bulbs. Steep for 12 hrs. Strain. Add sugar or honey to make consistency of syrup. Bruised and boiled caraway and sweet fennel seeds in vinegar will mask unpleasant smell of garlic. Use for coughs and asthma as needed.

C

PLANT IDENTIFICATION #5

RED CLOVER

Meadow Clover, Bee-Bread
Trefoil, Cow Clover

TRIFOLIUM PRATENSE

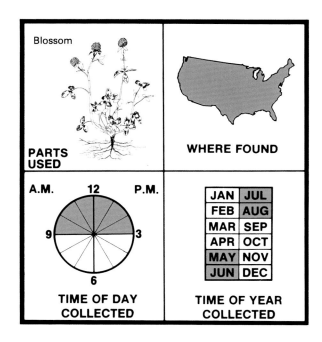

Blossom **PARTS USED**	**WHERE FOUND**
A.M. 12 P.M. 9 3 6 **TIME OF DAY COLLECTED**	JAN JUL FEB AUG MAR SEP APR OCT MAY NOV JUN DEC **TIME OF YEAR COLLECTED**

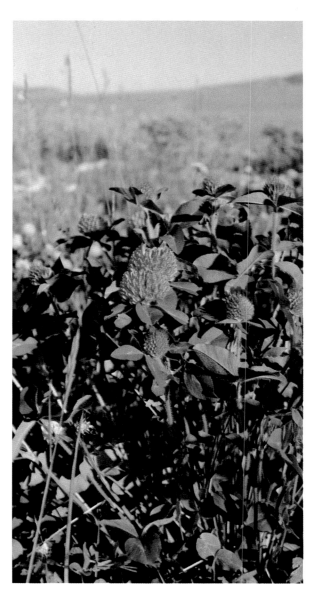

MEDICINAL USES:

- Relieves mental stress
- Purifies the blood
- Whooping cough

- Whooping cough

PLANT INFORMATION:

Red Clover is a member of the Pea Family (Leguminosae) and is found everywhere. The flower is the important part of this plant.

The infusion can be taken in place of coffee which will bring good purifying effects to the blood stream.

Collect in the summer month and dry in a semi-shady area. Store in a vermin-proof bag or container for use in the winter.

Clover and alfalfa (same family) is a good source of Vitamin B_{17}.

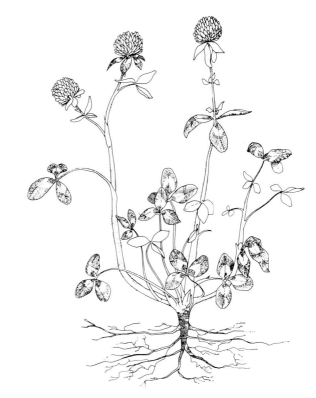

PREPARATION:

INFUSION (See Section 7 for General Infusion Preparation Information)

STANDARD INFUSION

Take freely - Wineglassful doses

SYRUP (Special Preparation)

1 oz. dried flower heads added to 1 pint sugar water (simple sugar). Boil and strain.

Take freely as needed.

MEDICINAL PROPERTIES

Antispasmodic
Demulcent
Sedative
Antitussive
Alterative

COMBINATIONS

for Purifying
the Blood
{ Equal Parts
Red Clover
Burdock
Blue Flag }
Standard
Infusion
Drink Freely

PLANT MORPHOLOGY

Plant Morphology is the study of plant form or structure (*Morpho* = form + *ology* = the study of). Botanists analyze plant structures to identify and classify plants. The general shape of the plant, size, color, and other physical characteristics are observed. When "keying out" a plant (see page 150) various plant parts are compared to determine structure similarities and differences so that the exact plant species may be determined. The flower is the most important plant structure used in identifying plants. Flower shape, color, number of petals and sepals, positions of the female parts of the flower, etc. are important characteristics. Other structures, such as flower and leaf arrangement on the stems, growth habitat, pubescense and leaf margins are also used.

There are three basic flower shapes:

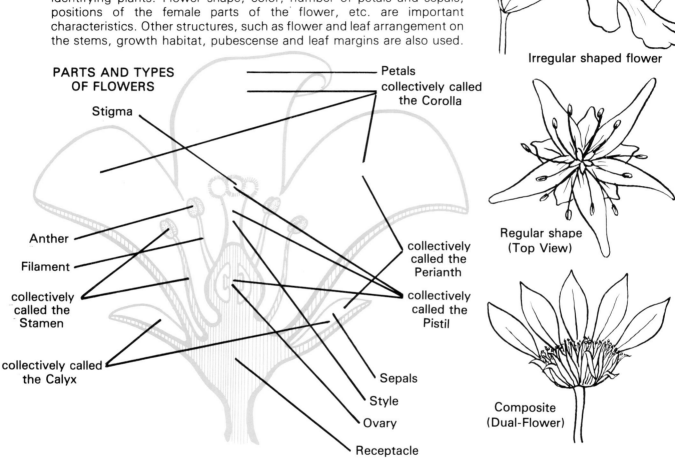

PARTS AND TYPES OF FLOWERS

Petals collectively called the Corolla

Stigma

Anther

Filament

collectively called the Stamen

collectively called the Calyx

collectively called the Perianth

collectively called the Pistil

Sepals

Style

Ovary

Receptacle

Irregular shaped flower

Regular shape (Top View)

Composite (Dual-Flower)

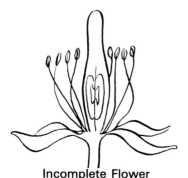

Incomplete Flower
(Missing one or more floral parts)

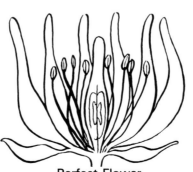

Perfect Flower
(Has both Male and Female parts - Pistils and Stamens)

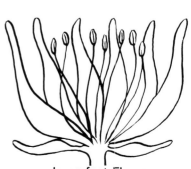

Imperfect Flower
(Lacking either Pistils or Stamens)

Position of the Ovary in the Flower

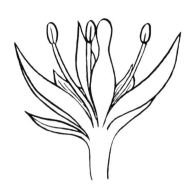

Hypogynous
Ovary Superior to the floral cup

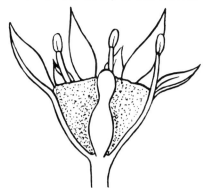

Perigynous
Ovary Superior - surrounded by floral cup.

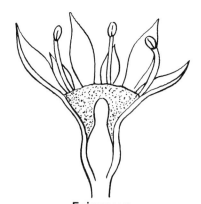

Epigynous
Ovary Inferior - Ovary appears
to be in the flower stem.

Arrangement of Flowers on the stem (Inflorescence)

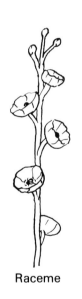

Raceme

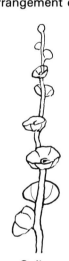

Spike

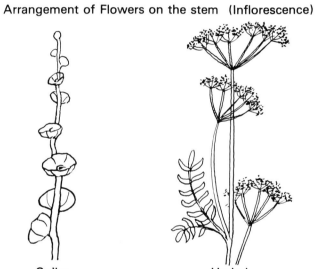

Umbel

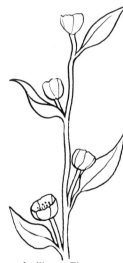

Axillary Flowers

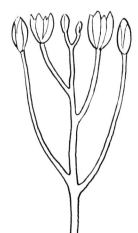

A Corymb

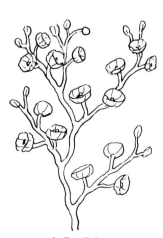

A Panicle

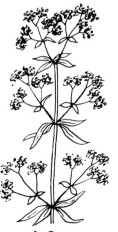

A Cyme

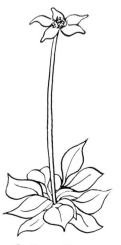

Solitary Flower

31

Arrangement of Leaves on the Stems

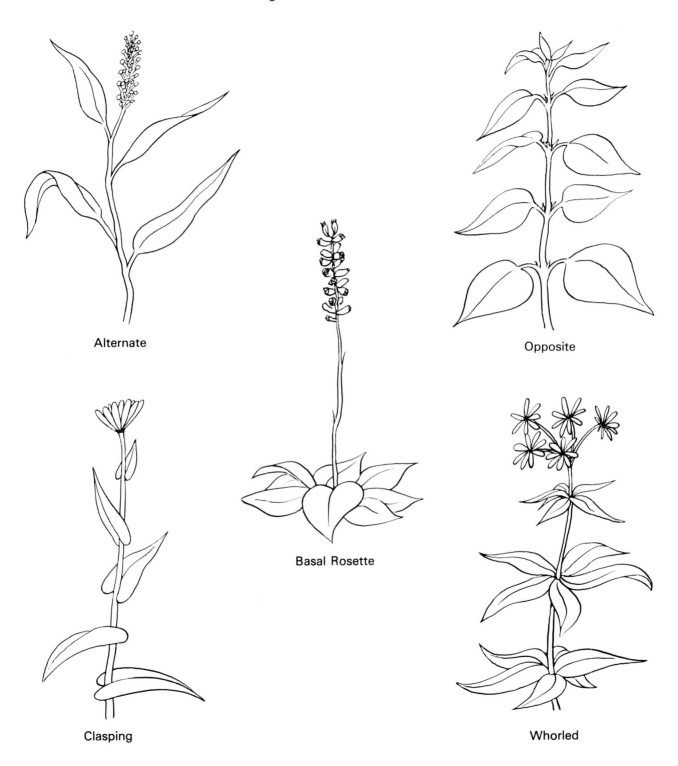

Alternate

Opposite

Basal Rosette

Clasping

Whorled

Types and Shapes of Leaves

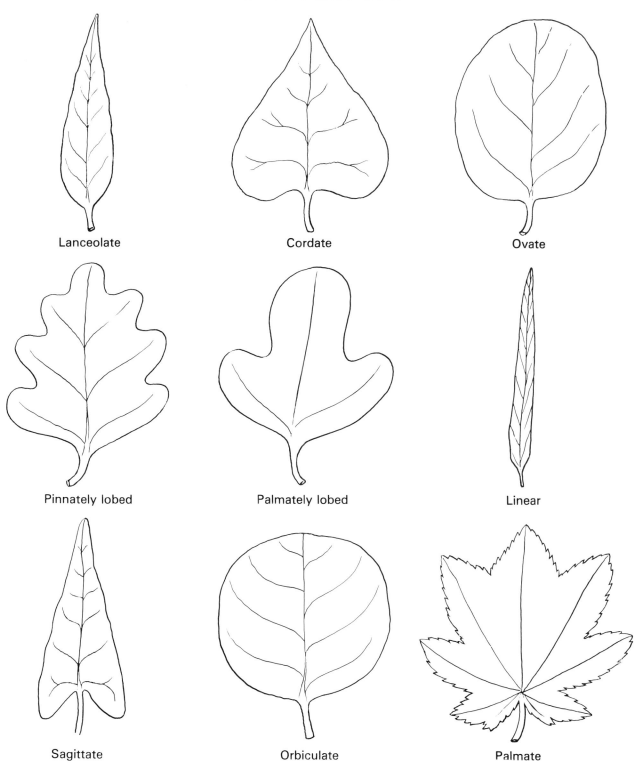

Lanceolate

Cordate

Ovate

Pinnately lobed

Palmately lobed

Linear

Sagittate

Orbiculate

Palmate

Root Systems

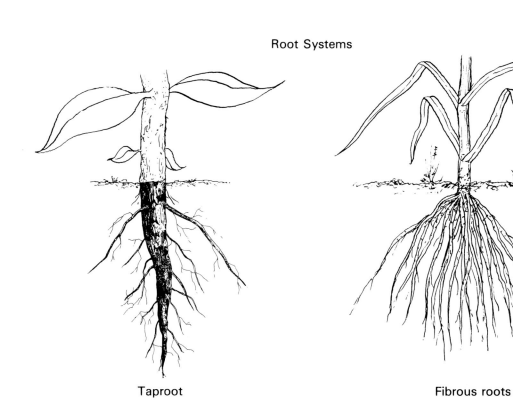

Taproot

Fibrous roots

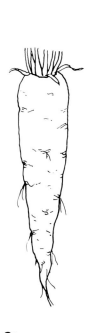

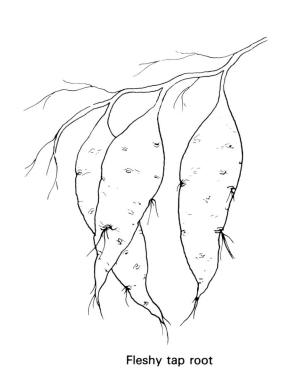

Storage root

Fleshy tap root

Section II

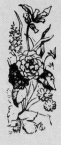

Spearmint

The Meadow Enhancer

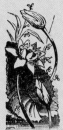

Peppermint

The Rodent Chaser

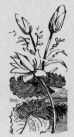

Catnip

The Feline Fascinator

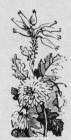

Horsemint

Montezuma's Placator

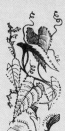

Pennyroyal

The Anti-seizure Plant

PLANT IDENTIFICATION #6

SPEARMINT
Garden Mint, Green Mint
Fish Mint, Lamb Mint
Mackerel Mint, Spire Mint

MENTHA VIRIDIS
Mentha spicata

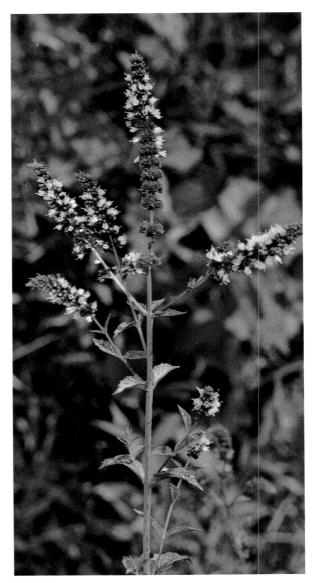

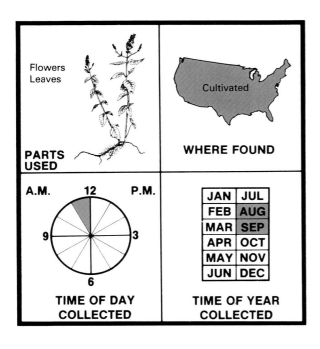

Flowers Leaves	**Cultivated**
PARTS USED	**WHERE FOUND**
A.M. 12 P.M. 9 3 6	JAN JUL / FEB AUG / MAR SEP / APR OCT / MAY NOV / JUN DEC
TIME OF DAY COLLECTED	**TIME OF YEAR COLLECTED**

MEDICINAL USES:

- Gas in stomach & bowels
- Dyspepsia
- Spasms
- Dropsy
- Gravel in bladder
- Piles (injection)

- Vomiting during pregnancy
- Dysuria
- Suppressed urine

PLANT INFORMATION:

Spearmint is in the Mint Family (Labiatae) and has a wide distribution in the U.S. It grows mostly in heavy clay-loam soil near springs and river banks.

All of the Mints should be collected from areas which are partially shaded by a bush or a tree canopy. Mints collected under partial shade have higher amounts of oil in their leaves than those growing in open sunlight or in the shadows.

Spearmint is generally less potent than the peppermints, and may be better adapted for childrens doses.

When collecting the mints for drying and storing purposes, cut the stem 2 or 3 inches above the ground and tie loosely into bunches. Hang tied plants in a warm, dry, indirectly lighted area.

Place dried herbs in an airtight container because they are very hygroscopic.

Never boil the mints as it will destroy their medicinal contents.

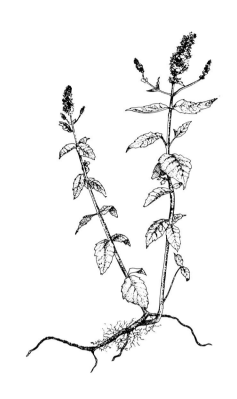

PREPARATION:

INFUSION (See Section 7 for General Infusion Preparation Information)

STANDARD INFUSION

Dosage: 1 cupful B.I.D. Morning and evening

TINCTURE (See Section 6 for General Tincture Preparation Information)

Gather leaves and flowering heads and place in ½ qt. jar. Add enough Gin to cover herb and soak for 7 days. Express, filter, bottle.

Dosage: 10 to 50 minums in hot water B.I.D.

MEDICINAL PROPERTIES

Carminative
Stimulant
Diaphoretic
Diuretic
Antispasmodic

COMBINATIONS

Colic & Cramps { Spearmint Horehound } Standard Tincture 10 drops B.I.D.

PLANT IDENTIFICATION #7

PEPPERMINT
Brandy Mint
White Mint
Balm Mint

MENTHA PIPERITA

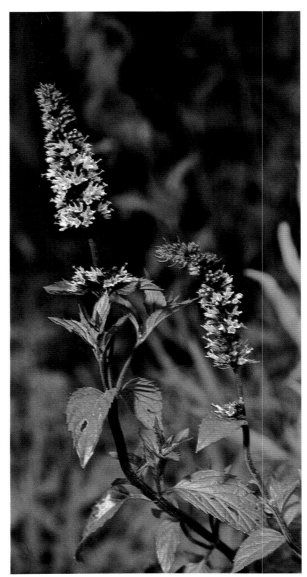

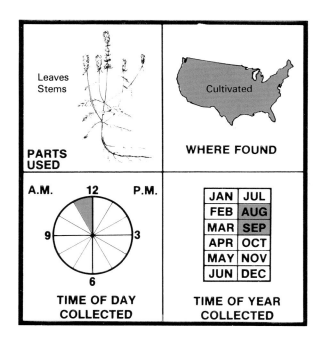

Leaves Stems **PARTS USED**	**WHERE FOUND** — Cultivated
A.M. 12 **P.M.** 9 · 3 6 **TIME OF DAY COLLECTED**	JAN / JUL FEB / AUG MAR / SEP APR / OCT MAY / NOV JUN / DEC **TIME OF YEAR COLLECTED**

MEDICINAL USES:

• Insomnia • Colic • Flatulence • Dysentery • Vomiting • Headache	• Infection • Toothache	• Colic • Flatulence • Palpitation of the heart	• Colic • Flatulence

PLANT INFORMATION:

Peppermint is in the Mint Family (Labiatae).

Given equal quantities and quality, Peppermint is more potent than Spearmint. A general rule for using these plants is: Peppermint for the adult, and Spearmint for the child.

A key identifying characteristic of the mint family is that the stems are square.

If you plan to cultivate this plant, do not use the same soil for more than two consecutive years for the soil will not support the nutritional requirements beyond this period.

Peppermint oil is violently disliked by rats and can be useful in their eradication.

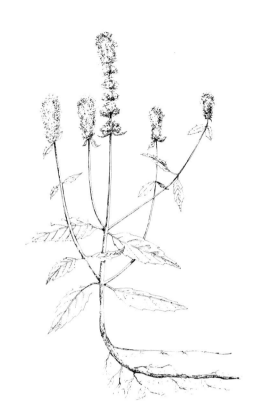

PREPARATION:

INFUSION (See Section 7 for General Infusion Preparation Information)

STANDARD INFUSION

Dosage: Wineglassful, frequently as needed

FLUID EXTRACT (See Section 6 for General Extraction Preparation Information)

STANDARD FLUID EXTRACT

Dosage: ¼ to 1 drachm T.I.D.

TINCTURE (See Section 6 for General Tincture Preparation Information)

STANDARD TINCTURE

Dosage: 5 to 20 drops T.I.D.

Commercial Oil *

COMBINATIONS:

MEDICINAL PROPERTIES								
Antiseptic Carminative Nervine Stomachic	Teething Children	{	½ oz. Peppermint ½ oz. Scullcap ½ oz. Pennyroyal	}	Standard Infusion Strain Sweeten	Cold or Flu	{ Peppermint Yarrow Elderberry Flowers }	Standard Infusion of Equal parts

*NOTE: The oils of Spearmint, Peppermint, Horsemint, Catnep and Pennyroyal can be obtained from Royal Botanical Company, P.O. Box 2054, Pocatello, Idaho 83201.

PLANT IDENTIFICATION #8

CATNEP

Catnip, Catmint
Catrup, Field Balm
Cats Wort

NEPETA CATARIA

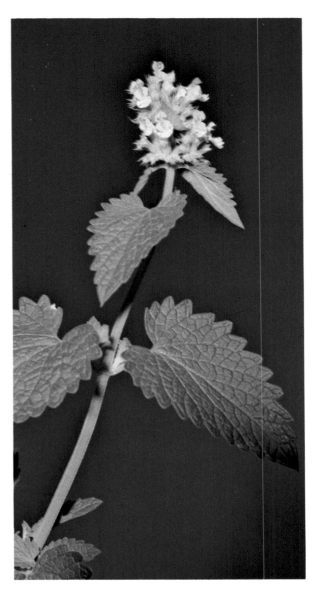

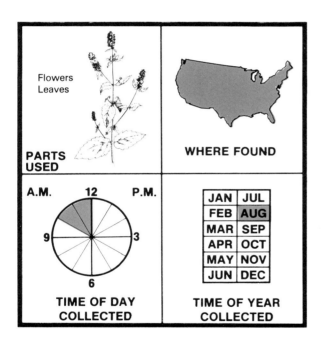

Flowers Leaves **PARTS USED**	**WHERE FOUND**
A.M. 12 **P.M.** 9 3 6 **TIME OF DAY COLLECTED**	JAN / JUL FEB / **AUG** MAR / SEP APR / OCT MAY / NOV JUN / DEC **TIME OF YEAR COLLECTED**

MEDICINAL USES:

- Fever

- Stomach acid

- Colic

- Flatulence

- Produces urination
  where it has stopped

- Fever

- Stomach acid

- Colic

- Flatulence

- Produces urination
  where it has stopped

PLANT INFORMATION:

Catnep is in the Mint Family (Labiatae). The name is derived from the fact that cats have a strange fascination for the plant and, if bruised, will try to destroy it.

Folklore records that chewing the root will produce personality changes — from a meek, docile individual — to a fierce, courageous person.

The smell of catnep resembles the smell of Pennyroyal and Peppermint.

Catnep will produce perspiration and is a functional treatment for colds and fevers.

It makes a refreshing substitute for our more common commercial teas.

The tea should never be boiled.

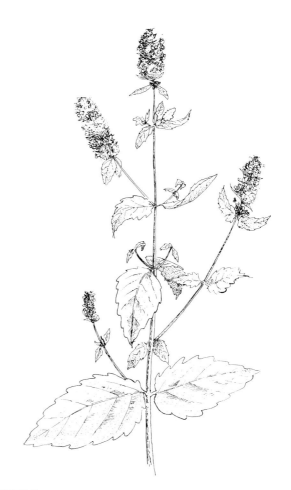

PREPARATION:

INFUSION (See Section 7 for General Infusion Preparation Information)

STANDARD INFUSION

Dosage: Adult - 2 tablespoonsful Q.I.D.
Children - 2 or 3 teaspoonsful T.I.D.

TINCTURE (See Section 6 for General Tincture Preparation Information)

STANDARD TINCTURE

Dosage: 5 to 20 drops T.I.D.

MEDICINAL PROPERTIES

Anodyne, Antispasmodic
Carminative, Aromatic
Diaphoretic, Nervine
Refrigerant

COMBINATIONS:

Scarlet Fever and Small Pox { Saffron Catnep } Equal parts Standard Infusion

PLANT IDENTIFICATION #9

HORSEMINT

Spotted Monarda
Bergamont
Bee Balm

Monarda punctata
Monarda lutea
Monarda didyma
Monarda fistulosa

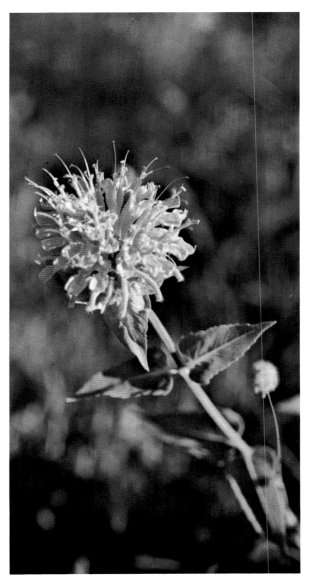

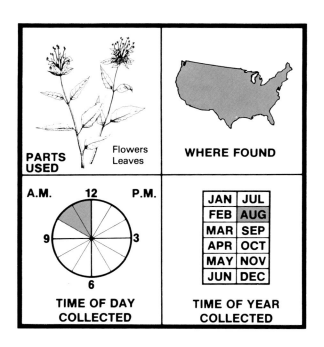

| PARTS USED | Flowers Leaves | WHERE FOUND |
| TIME OF DAY COLLECTED | | TIME OF YEAR COLLECTED |

A.M. 12 P.M.
9 3
6

JAN	JUL
FEB	AUG
MAR	SEP
APR	OCT
MAY	NOV
JUN	DEC

MEDICINAL USES:

- Colds

- Diarrhea

- Stomach gas

- Colic

- Rheumatism

- Colds

- Diarrhea

- Stomach gas

- Colic

PLANT INFORMATION:

This plant is named after the 16th Century plant physician, Nicolas Monardes, of Seville, Spain.

It readily yields its medicinal virtues to an infusion, but the oil yields even better to an alcohol tincture.

The oil of Horsemint is useful in treating rheumatism or where other rubefacients are indicated.

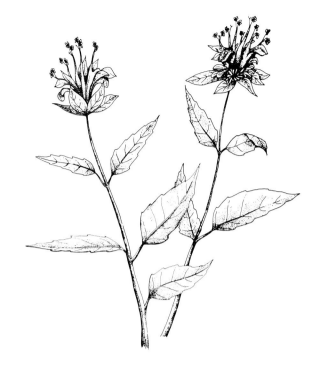

PREPARATION:

INFUSION (See Section 7 for General Infusion Preparation Information)

STANDARD INFUSION

Dosage: 1 capful B.I.D. Morning and Evening

OIL (Special Preparation)

COMMERCIALLY OBTAINED

TINCTURE (See Section 6 for General Tincture Preparation Information)

Gather leaves and flowering heads. Place in ½ qt. jar, add enough (Holland) Gin to cover herb, soak for seven days. Express, filter, bottle and cork.

Dosage: 10 to 50 minims in hot water B.I.D.

MEDICINAL PROPERTIES

Carminative
Diuretic
Stimulant
Diaphoretic
Rubefacient

PLANT IDENTIFICATION #10

PENNYROYAL

Pulegium, Squawmint
American Pennyroyal
Run-by-the-Ground
Lurk-in-the-Ditch, Tickweed
Mosquito plant, Pudding grass

HEDEOMA PULEGIOIDES (AMERICAN)
Mentha pulegium (English)

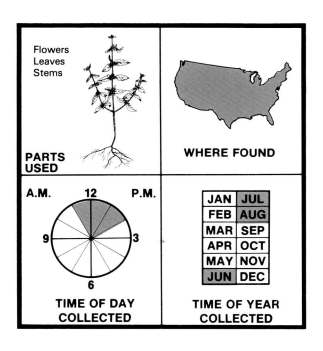

Flowers Leaves Stems **PARTS USED**	**WHERE FOUND**
A.M. 12 P.M. 9 · 3 6 **TIME OF DAY COLLECTED**	JAN JUL FEB AUG MAR SEP APR OCT MAY NOV JUN DEC **TIME OF YEAR COLLECTED**

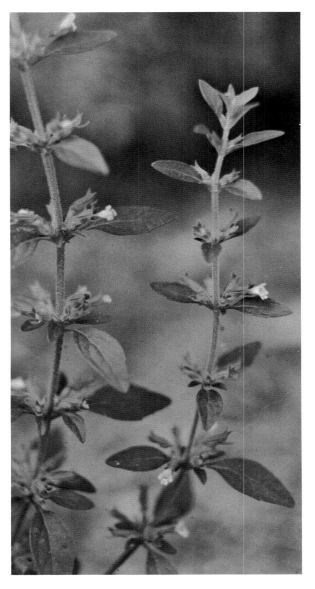

MEDICINAL USES:

• Epilepsy	• Epilepsy	• Epilepsy
• Colds	• Colds	• Colds
• Flu	• Flu	• Flu
• Fever	• Fever	• Fever
• Jaundice	• Jaundice	• Jaundice
• Lack of Perspiration	• Lack of Perspiration	• Lack of Perspiration
• Colic	• Colic	• Colic
• Gas on Stomach	• Gas on Stomach	• Gas on Stomach

PLANT INFORMATION:

Pennyroyal is in the Mint Family (Labiatae). The oil should never be used by pregnant women and the dosage should be well regulated to stay within the recommended dosages.

By crushing the tender leaves and rubbing it on the exposed surfaces of the skin, it can be used externally to repel insects.

Pennyroyal has many uses.

When cultivating the pennyroyal, select the American genus, for it can withstand the colder North American climate.

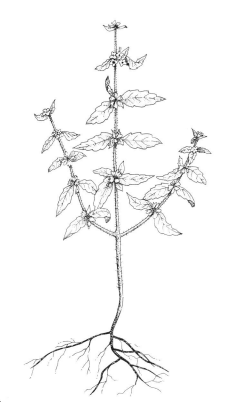

PREPARATION:

INFUSION (See Section 7 for General Infusion Preparation Information)

STANDARD INFUSION

Dosage: One teacupful T.I.D.

POWDER (See Section 8 for General Powder Preparation Information)

Dosage: 30 to 50 gr. B.I.D.

TINCTURE (See Section 6 for General Tincture Preparation Information)

STANDARD TINCTURE

Dosage: ½ to 1 fluid drahm B.I.D.

MEDICINAL PROPERTIES
Carminative
Diaphoretic
Insect Repellant
Antispasmodic

MINT IDENTIFICATION:

The Mints (Labiatae) are identified by their aromatic scent, and structurally by their square stems. The petals (Corolla) are united forming a tube which forms two "lips" on the outward part, hence the name, Labiate, or Lips.

It is a large family with about 150 genera and over 3000 species. It is almost cosmopolitan in distribution, but it seldom grows in the arctic or alpine regions.

The plant illustrations shown below will help identify and differentiate between the mints listed in this section, and some of the other mints you will see in the field.

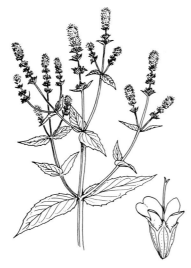

Mentha spicata

Spearmint is a perennial mint which grows from creeping rhizomes.

The leaves are sessile or spiked (attached to stem without a leaf petiole)

Stamens: 4
Flower color: Pale lavender to White
Availability: June - August

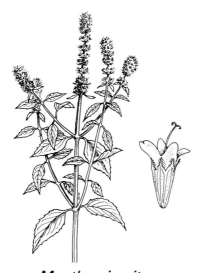

Mentha piperita

Peppermint is a perennial mint which also grows from underground stems (rhizomes).

The leaves are petiolate. (Lanceolate-ovate to elliptic)

Flowers crowded in a dense terminal spike.
Stamens: 4
Flower color: Pink Lavender to White
Availability: July - September

Horsemint generally grows on a singular stem with one or several dense terminal flower heads.

The leaves are toothed and the plant is mostly perennial. The corolla is 3-lobed.

The plant is named after the Spanish Physician and Botanist (Nicolas Monardes).

Stamens: 2
Flower Color: Pink - Purple
Availability: June - August

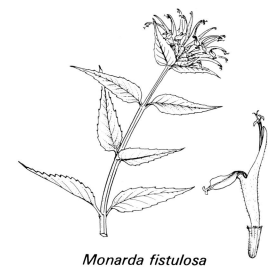

Monarda fistulosa

Catnep is a taprooted perennial. It has commonly 3 or more stems per plant.

Corolla 2-lipped.
Stamens: 4
Flower Color: Whitish-dotted with purple
　　　　　　　　rarely yellow.
Availability: June - September

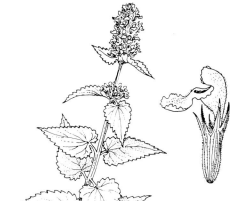

Nepeta cataria

Penneyroyal is annual or can be perennial Grows in dry open places (in lower elevation).

Corolla Bilabiate
Stamens: 2
Flower Color: Light Purple
Availability: June - August

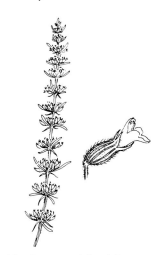

Hedeoma hispidum

FIELD NOTES/LABORATORY NOTES

Section III

**Five Botanicals
Collecting, Drying and
Storage of Botanicals**

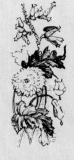

Plantago

The Contingency Plant

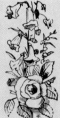

Rose Hips

The Health Guardians

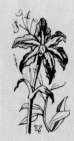

Oregon Grape

Mountain Lovers Companion

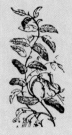

Shave Grass

The Renal Rejuvinator

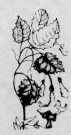

Juniper Berries

The Pancreatic Pal

PLANT IDENTIFICATION #11

PLANTAGO

Cuckoo's Bread, Waybread,
Englishman's Foot, Rattail,
Chimney Sweep, Bird Seed,
Devil's Shoestring, Ribgrass,
White Man's Foot, Snakeweed.

PLANTAGO MAJOR

Plantago lanceolata
Plantago ovata
Plantago psyllium
Plantago species

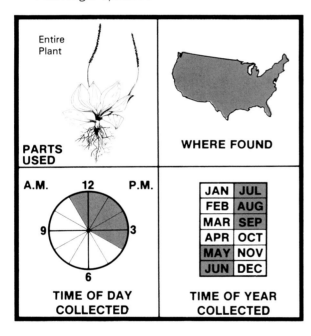

Entire Plant **PARTS USED**	**WHERE FOUND**
A.M. 12 P.M. 9 3 6 **TIME OF DAY COLLECTED**	JAN JUL / FEB AUG / MAR SEP / APR OCT / MAY NOV / JUN DEC **TIME OF YEAR COLLECTED**

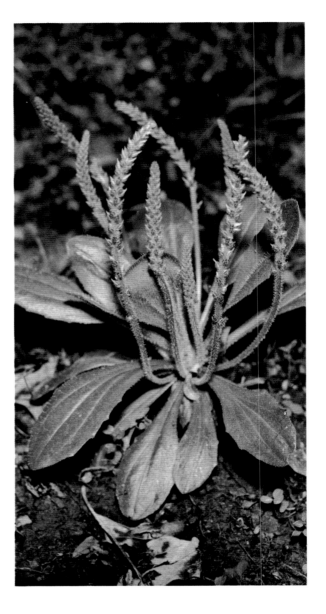

MEDICINAL USES:

- Boils
- Carbuncles
- Pink eye
- Insect and Snake Bites
- Blood poisoning
- Hemostatic
- Staphylococcus infections
- Eczema

- Leucorrhea (Whites) (Vaginal Injection)
- Frog or Thrush in Children (Gargle)
- Excessive mucus production (Drink)
- Diarrhea (Drink)

- Hemorrhoids
- Impetigo
- Staphylococcus infections

PLANT INFORMATION:

Plantago is a member of the Plantain Family (Plantaginaceae). It is a common lawn pest, but is one of the best medicinal plants available to the herbalist.

Its active antiseptic properties equals or surpasses some of the best commercial antibiotics.

Plantago can be used either freshly picked or dried and powdered.

For treating conjunctivitis (Pink-eye), a warm poultice may be applied directly to the closed, infected eye. A standard infusion using distilled water may be effectively used as a wash.

The seeds are laxative. Soak about one gram of the seeds (especially of the Eastern species *Plantago psyllium*) in 20cc of distilled water for about 24 hours. Take plenty of water with each 8 gram dose.

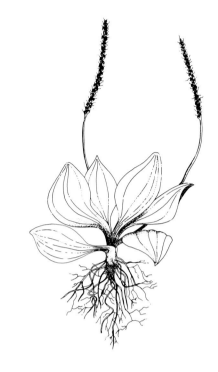

PREPARATION:

INFUSION (See Section 7 for General Infusion Preparation Information)

STANDARD INFUSION

As indicated or needed

POULTICE (See Section 4 for General Poultice Preparation Information)

STANDARD POULTICE

As needed

OINTMENT (See Section 5 for General Ointment Preparation Information)

STANDARD OINTMENT

(For Hemorrhoids: Slowly boil 2 ounces of contused leaves in peanut or safflower oil for 2 hours. Apply to affected area as needed.)

MEDICINAL PROPERTIES

Antiseptic
Demulcent
Alterative
Vulnerary
Diuretic
Emmenogogue
Astringent

PLANT IDENTIFICATION #12

ROSE HIPS

ROSA RUGOSA
  Rosa woodsii
  Rosa nutkana
  Rosa multiflora
  Rosa species

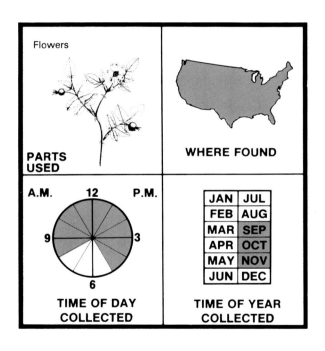

Flowers **PARTS USED**	**WHERE FOUND**
A.M. 12 P.M. 9 3 6 **TIME OF DAY COLLECTED**	JAN JUL / FEB AUG / MAR SEP / APR OCT / MAY NOV / JUN DEC **TIME OF YEAR COLLECTED**

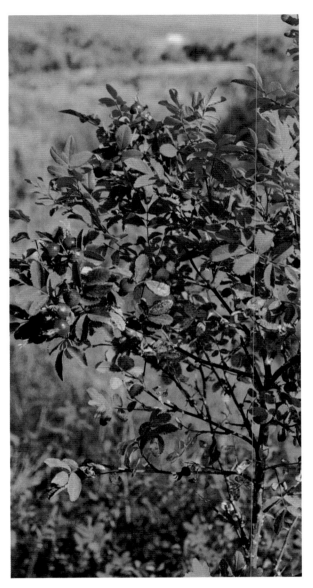

MEDICINAL USES:

- Nutritional benefits
- Colds
- Arteriosclerosis
- Vitamin C source
- Nutritional jam

PLANT INFORMATION:

As the name "Rose-hip" reveals, this plant is in the Rose Family (Rosaceae). Rose-hips are medicinal from a vitamin-nutritional point-of-view.

They are very widespread throughout the U.S. and easy to collect and store for future use.

It is the fleshy edible vegetative floral receptacle which contains the Vitamin C. Each average size "hip" contains between 350 and 500 milligrams of Vitamin C.

There are many species of this plant, all of which contain the C Vitamin. Cultivated Roses can be used, but the wild varieties are a better source.

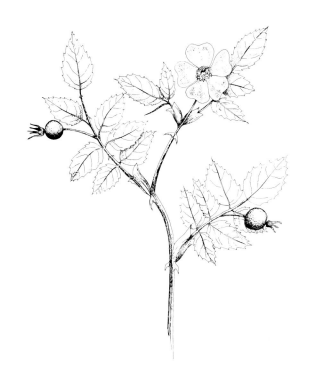

PREPARATION:

INFUSION (See Section 7 for General Infusion Preparation Information)

STANDARD INFUSION

Sweeten with honey and drink either hot or cold.

Dosage: Drink freely.

Rose-Hip Jam:

NOTE: Avoid the use of aluminum cookery.

Place four pounds of freshly collected and washed rose-hips into a stainless steel or porcelain cooker. Add five cups of cold water. Heat to a boil. Boil for 15 minutes. Press and strain through a sturdy muslin cloth into a saucepan. Add one whole lime or one-half lemon, and one pound of sugar and one-fourth pound light honey to each two pounds of the strained hips. Mix well.

Heat at a low temperature for 25 to 30 minutes. Stir frequently. When jam begins to simmer vigorously, continue heat for 10 more minutes. Place in mason jars and seal as you do your regular canning.

**MEDICINAL
PROPERTIES**
Antiscorbutic

PLANT IDENTIFICATION #13

OREGON GRAPE

MAHONIA AQUIFOLIUM
  Mahonia repens
  Mahonia bealei
  Mahonia fremontii

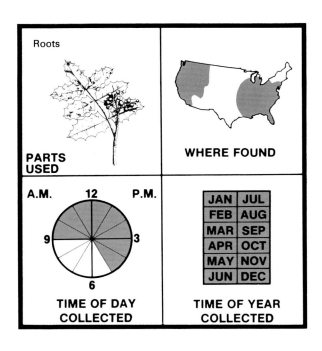

Roots

PARTS USED

WHERE FOUND

A.M. 12 P.M.

9   3

6

TIME OF DAY COLLECTED

JAN	JUL
FEB	AUG
MAR	SEP
APR	OCT
MAY	NOV
JUN	DEC

TIME OF YEAR COLLECTED

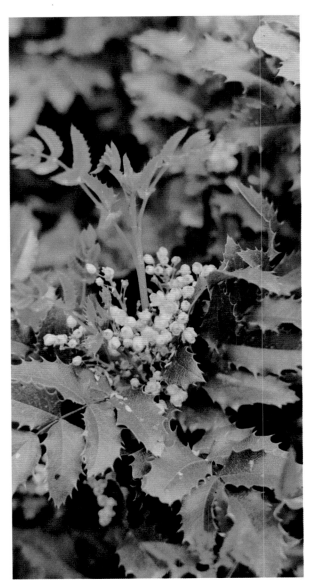

MEDICINAL USES:

- Blood purifyer
- Eliminates catabolic wastes
- Herpes
- Eczema
- Psoriasis

- Diseased genitals
- Catarrahal disorders of the stomach, intestines and renal-cystic organs.

PLANT INFORMATION:

This evergreen plant is in the Barberry Family (Berberidaceae). Some botanists list the genus as Mahonia, while others prefer to name the genus Berberis.

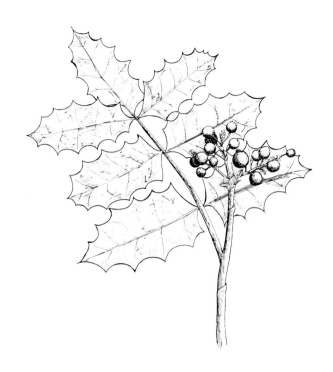

Oregon grape can be collected in the West and in the East. There are four main species with the same basic medicinal values, namely; *Mahonia repens* (the low or creeping type), *Mahonia aquifolium* (the best one to use, and the one cultivated mainly as a landscape ornamental), *Mahonia bealei* (also cultivated), and *Mahonia fremontii* (a southern species) a small, stout, prickly blue-leaved plant.

It can be collected in every month of the year - weather conditions permitting.

The root contains the active medicinal properties.

PREPARATION:

INFUSION (See Section 7 for General Infusion Preparation Information)
STANDARD INFUSION
Dosage: 1 to 4 fluid ounces T.I.D.

POWDERED PLANT (See Section 8 for General Powdering Preparation Information)
Powder and capsulate in 5 to 20 grains
Dosage: 1 to 4 capsules daily for one week

MEDICINAL PROPERTIES
Alterative
Tonic
Detergent
Digestant

PLANT IDENTIFICATION #14

SHAVE GRASS
Horsetail, Scouring Rush
Bottle Brush, Paddock-Pipes
Pewterwort, Joint Grass

EQUISETUM ARVENSE
Equisetum hymenale

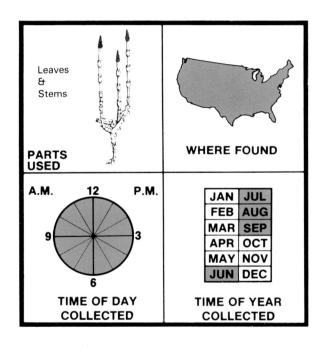

Leaves & Stems

PARTS USED

WHERE FOUND

A.M.   12   P.M.
9   3
6

TIME OF DAY COLLECTED

JAN	JUL
FEB	AUG
MAR	SEP
APR	OCT
MAY	NOV
JUN	DEC

TIME OF YEAR COLLECTED

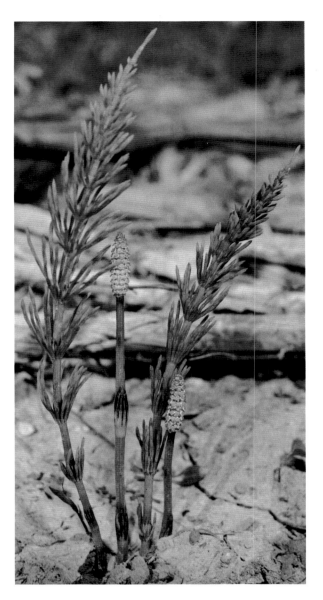

MEDICINAL USES:

- Foul-smelling Sores

- Nephritis (with edema)
- Prostatic conditions of the aged
- Passive bleeding of the kidney
- Inflamed renal mucosa
- Aides in passing gravel or stones

- Dysuria
- Nephritis (with edema)
- Prostatic conditions of the aged
- Passive bleeding of the kidney
- Inflamed mucosa
- Prevent and rids gravel or stones

PLANT INFORMATION:

Shave grass is in the Horsetail Family (Equisetaceae). Botanically speaking, it is a very primitive plant being found as fossils in rocks dating back to the Paleozoic Era. They first developed during the Devonian times and reached their climax during the Mississippian time period with some species growing over thirty feet tall. In fact one tropical species of "Horsetail" grows to the same height today.

Besides its therapeutic value, it also makes an excellent abrasive "scouring rush" agent for out-of-door cleaning of pots and pans. This is due to its high content of silica which gives the plant its course gritty texture.

It is found and collected in two forms (see picture on the adjacent page.) One - the slender, tall stem with a spore bearing strobilus, and Two - a sterile branch with a whorl of branchlets at each node, resembling a "horse tail".

Joint-grass, another name attached to this plant, is found growing along river banks and in other damp areas. It can also thrive in comparatively dry meadows and even on railroad embankments.

It is not a grass.

MEDICINAL PROPERTIES
Astringent
Antiseptic
Tonic
Diuretic
Emmenogogue
Homestatic

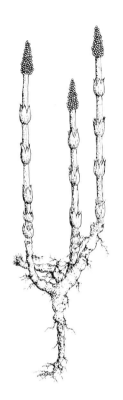

PREPARATION:

POULTICE (See Section 4 for General Poultice Preparation Information)

STANDARD POULTICE

Dosage: As needed.

INFUSION (See Section 7 for General Infusion Preparation Information)

STANDARD INFUSION

Dosage: One to four cups daily for 4 to 6 days. Repeat at 3 week intervals.

TINCTURE (See Section 6 for General Tincture Preparation Information)

STANDARD TINCTURE

Dosage: 5 to 40 minims

PLANT IDENTIFICATION #15

JUNIPER BERRIES
Common Juniper
Mountain Red Juniper
Utah Juniper
Cedar Berries

JUNIPERUS COMMUNIS
Juniperus scopulorum
Juniperus utahensis
Juniperus species

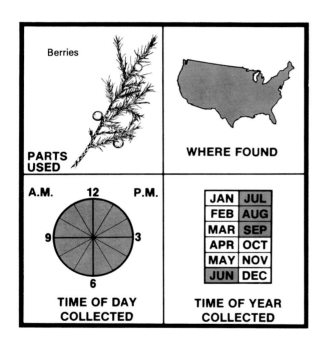

Berries

PARTS USED

WHERE FOUND

A.M.	12	P.M.

9   3

6

TIME OF DAY COLLECTED

JAN	JUL
FEB	AUG
MAR	SEP
APR	OCT
MAY	NOV
JUN	DEC

TIME OF YEAR COLLECTED

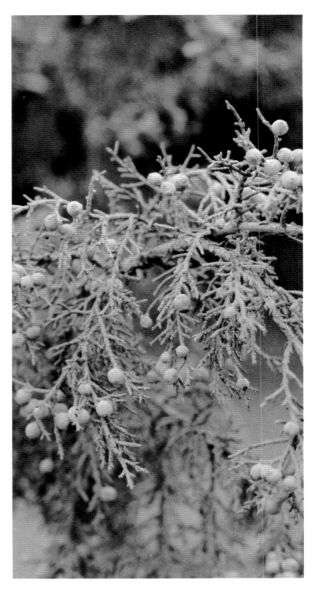

MEDICINAL USES:

- Renal Catarrh
- Gleet
- Diabetes
- Scorbutic Diseases
- Gargle when exposed to contagious disease

- Hypoglycemia
- Adrenal dysfunction
- Pancreas dysfunction

PLANT INFORMATION:

Juniper is a member of the Cypress Family (Cupressaceae) which also includes other flora as the Arbor Vitae, Incense Cedar, Port Orford Cedar, and the Everglades Cypress. None of these are true cedars *(Cedrus)* which are actually in the Pine Family *Pinaceae.*

Two tree-like species of native western Junipers, - the Utah Juniper, *Juniperus utahensis var. osteosperma,* and the Mt. Red Juniper, *Juniperus scopulorum* are commonly called ''cedar'' and in the West have long been used for making fence posts.

Most of the shrub-type Junipers are used for landscape ornamentals. All the berries are effective, the wild mountain juniper *Juniperus communis* is preferred.

It has a wide distribution in the western U.S. and extends into Canada and Alaska.

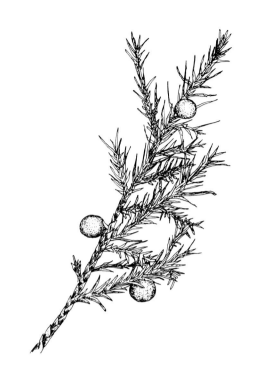

PREPARATION:

INFUSION (See Section 7 for General Infusion Preparation Information)

Soak 3 or 4 tablespoonsful of the berries for about one-half hour - in cold water. Steep in boiling water for another half hour. Cool.

Dosage: 3 or 4 cups daily.

TINCTURE (See Section 6 for General Tincture Preparation Information)

Macerate 1 ounce of the washed berries in 40% Ethyl Alcohol for 8 days.

Dosage: 15 to 30 drops in a large glass of water T.I.D.

MEDICINAL PROPERTIES

Antiscorbutic
Diuretic
Tonic
Antiseptic

59

COLLECTION, DRYING AND PRESERVATION OF MEDICINAL PLANTS

1. The active medicinal principle or virtue of a plant varies with such physical and environmental factors as:

   Light
   Temperature
   Season and Seasonal Fluctuations
   Elevation
   Moisture, etc.

   The time of day must be considered for the same reason. Plant chemicals change as the basic plant physiology changes from morning to night. Most plants can be collected in the morning after the dew and other moisture has evaporated.

2. The plant should be dried as soon after collecting as possible to prevent mildew or fermentation, which alters the plant's medicinal properties.

3. Only healthy looking plant parts should be used. Brown, unhealthy or discolored plant parts should not be collected.

4. Collections should be made away from busy, populated areas. This will help insure your collected plants will be free from sprays, toxins, and other harmful substances which may have been absorbed into the plant tissues.

5. Most plant parts above the ground (bark, seeds, stems, leaves and fruits) need not be cleaned. Underground parts should be thoroughly washed to prevent dirt from becoming part of the plant preparation.

6. After the plant is completely dried it should be stored away from air, moisture, warm temperatures and light, all of which are factors that promote plant deterioration. Most dried plants are hygroscopic (absorb moisture from the air) and therefore need to be stored in air-tight containers.

7. When possible, the entire plant should be used as each part imparts an essential virtue to the total medicinal action. This is especially meaningful with annual plants.

8. Roots should be collected in the early spring before the vegetative growth process has begun, or in the fall when all vegetative growth has ceased.

9. When a dried plant is cool to the touch, it is not completely dry.

10. Drying temperatures and time of drying should be adjusted to the individual plant. Coarse plants may take considerably longer than fragile, tender plants. 32° to 39° Centigrade is called "gentle heat" and is considered optimum.

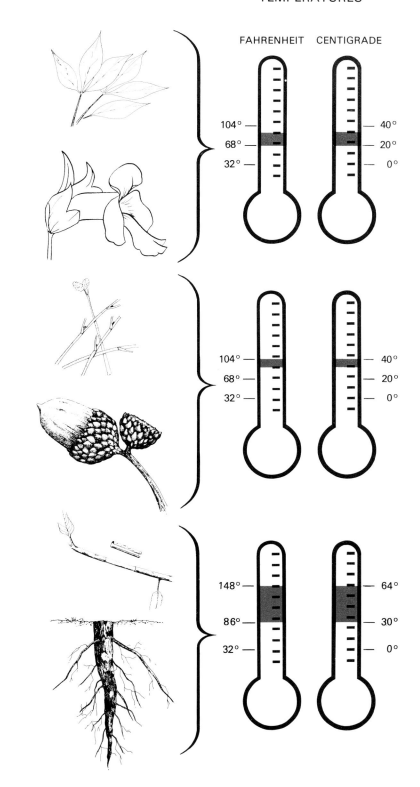

LEAVES

Collect when the flower is beginning to open.

FLOWERS

Collect just before flower is fully expanded.

STEMS (herbaceous)

Collect when the flower is beginning to open.

SEEDS AND FRUIT

Collect when fully ripe.

BARK

Collect in early spring or in the fall when all vegetative growth has ceased.

ROOTS

Collect in early spring or in the fall when all vegetative growth has ceased.

IDEAL DRYING
TEMPERATURES

FAHRENHEIT   CENTIGRADE

104°   40°
68°   20°
32°   0°

104°   40°
68°   20°
32°   0°

148°   64°
86°   30°
32°   0°

FIELD NOTES/LABORATORY NOTES

Section IV

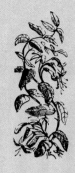

Life Root

The Womens Friend

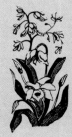

Tansey

The Hexapod Repeller

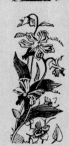

Burdock

The Rheumatic Healer

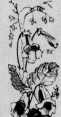

Arnica

The Naturo-physicians Friend

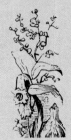

Golden Seal

The Universal Herb

PLANT IDENTIFICATION #16

LIFE ROOT

Squaw Weed
Ragwort
Female Regulator
Golden Senecio
Golden Ragwort

SENECIO AUREUS
Senecio vulgaris

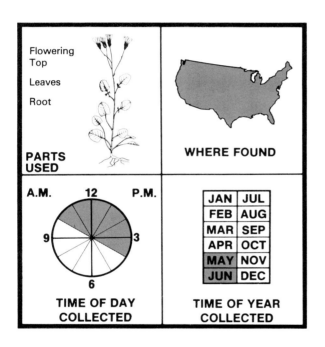

| Flowering Top Leaves Root **PARTS USED** | **WHERE FOUND** |

| **TIME OF DAY COLLECTED** | **TIME OF YEAR COLLECTED** |

JAN	JUL
FEB	AUG
MAR	SEP
APR	OCT
MAY	NOV
JUN	DEC

A.M. 12 P.M.
9   3
6

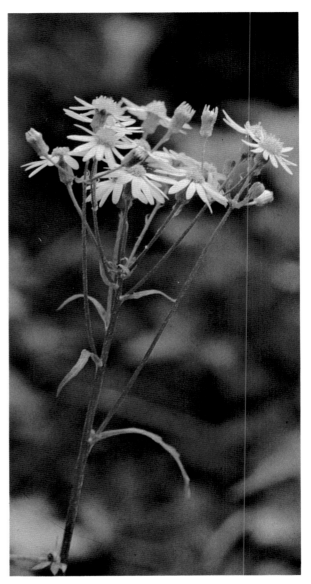

MEDICINAL USES:

- Dysmenorrhea
- Menorrhagia
- Atonic leukorrhea
- Prostate enlargement
- Functional irregularities (particularly during menopause)

- Dysmenorrhea
- Menorrhagia
- Atonic leukorrhea
- Prostate enlargement
- Functional irregularities (particularly during menopause)

PLANT INFORMATION:

This plant is a member of the Sunflower Family (Compositae). Its primary medicinal use is in treating female functional irregularities, especially during menopause.

It has stimulant effects to the pelvic plexus and will improve vascular activity in this region.

It has a strengthening effect to vaginal mucosa, adding tone to the flabby uterine ligaments caused by childbirth.

It tones the bladder, increasing its functional efficiency.

There is benefit in using it for painful menstuation and excessive uterine bleeding.

Life Root is safe to use.

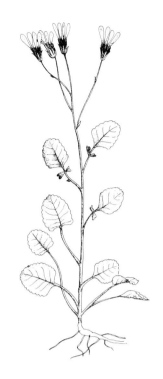

PREPARATION:

DECOCTION (See Section 7 for General Decoction Preparation Information)

Add 8 oz. roots to 16 oz. boiling water. Boil 3 to 10 minutes. Steep 10 minutes, strain and remove roots. Add amount of water lost to boiling. Add honey to sweeten.

Dosage: 2-8 fluid oz. daily.

TINCTURE (See Section 6 for General Tincture Preparation Information)

16 oz. green leaves. Add 1000cc. (32 oz.) alcohol (40%). Mix thoroughly. Macerate 14 days. Filter, bottle and cork.

Dosage: 10-25 minims (drops) in 8 oz. glass of water. B.I.D.

MEDICINAL PROPERTIES
Stimulant
Tonic
Diuretic
Emmenogogue

PLANT IDENTIFICATION #17

TANSEY

Bitter Buttons, Hindheel, Scent Fern
Ginger Plant, English Coat
Bachelor's Buttons, Parsley Fern

TANACETUM VULGARE

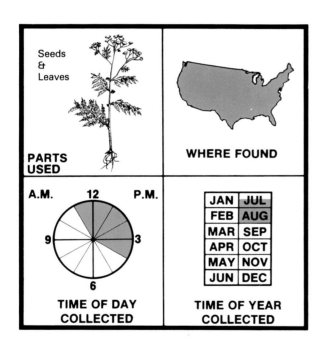

Seeds & Leaves **PARTS USED**	**WHERE FOUND**
A.M. 12 P.M. 9 3 6 **TIME OF DAY COLLECTED**	JAN JUL FEB AUG MAR SEP APR OCT MAY NOV JUN DEC **TIME OF YEAR COLLECTED**

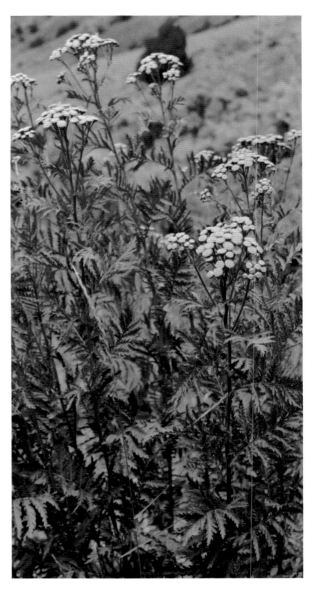

MEDICINAL USES:

- Expels worms (Pinworms)

- Painful menstration

- Insect repellant

66

PLANT INFORMATION:

Tansey is a member of the Sunflower Family (Compositae).

This plant should never be used by women who are pregnant. Internally its use should be under the direction of a physician. Overdoses (especially the Oil of Tansey) may be neurotoxic.

During the hunting season, Tansey leaves can be stripped from the stems and placed in a "Deer" or "Elk" bag to keep the flying insects away from the meat.

Rubbing the bruised leaves on the exposed body surfaces will also act as an insect repellent. A more permanent form can be made by bruising the leaves and soaking them in olive oil or a good mineral oil.

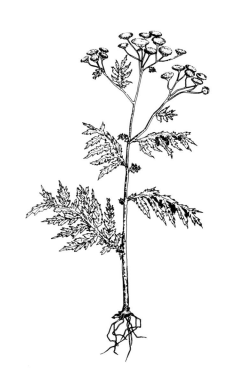

PREPARATION:

INFUSION (See Section 7 for General Infusion preparation information)

STANDARD INFUSION

Dosage: ½ to 1 wineglassful T.I.D. Reduced amounts for small children.

FIELD USE/Insect repellant

Crush leaves by rolling briskly between the palms of the hands. Rub on the exposed skin surfaces.

MEDICINAL PROPERTIES

Stimulant
Anthelminthic
Emmenagogic
Tonic

PLANT IDENTIFICATION #18

BURDOCK

Lappa, Thorny Burr
Begger's Buttons, Apersonata
Happy Major, Philanthropium
Cockelbur

ARCTIUM LAPPA L.
Arctium minus
Arctium species

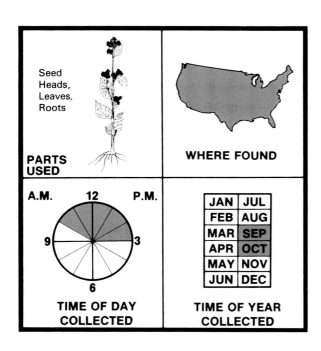

Seed Heads, Leaves, Roots

PARTS USED

WHERE FOUND

A.M.   12   P.M.

9   3

6

TIME OF DAY COLLECTED

JAN	JUL
FEB	AUG
MAR	SEP
APR	OCT
MAY	NOV
JUN	DEC

TIME OF YEAR COLLECTED

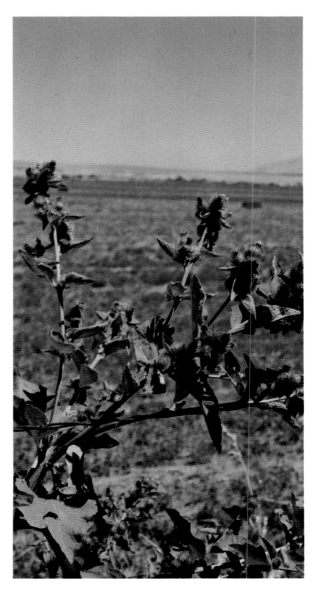

MEDICINAL USES:

• Arthritis	• Blood Diseases • Scurvy • Bladder and Kidney Disorders	• Cradle Cap • Eczema • Boils • Stys	• Blood Diseases • Scurvy • Bladder and Kidney Disorders

PLANT INFORMATION:

Burdock is in the Sunflower Family (Compositae) even though it shows little resemblance to what people generally think belongs to the Sunflowers. The fleshy roots from the first year's growth is the best to use.

The young stalks are edible if cut before the flower opens.

Use as a diuretic and renal tonic preparation when the kidney is malfunctioning in the following manner:

1) to clear the urine which is laden with mucus, pus cells, and red blood cells,

2) to aid in the expulsion of lithic material from the kidney and bladder, and

3) to soothe irritated Renal (kidney) and Cystic (bladder) mucosa.

Always take internally as teas in conjunction with topical applications when applicable.

Burdock is a good source of Vitamins A, C, B_2, B_3, and the minerals Iron, Calcium and Silicon.

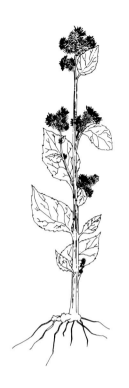

PREPARATION:

INFUSION (See Section 7 for General Infusion Preparation Information)

STANDARD INFUSION:

Dosage: 1 wineglassful T.I.D.

POULTICE (See Section 4 for General Poultice Preparation Information)

Bruise leaves and place on inflamed surface. Cover with hot, moist cloth.

DECOCTION (See Section 7 for General Decoction Preparation Information)

STANDARD DECOCTION

Dosage: 1 wineglassful T.I.D.

TINCTURE (See Section 6 for General Tincture Preparation Information)

Fill quart bottle with cocklebur. Add enough Vodka to fill jar. Macerate 3 days. Use out of jar until empty.

Dosage: 1 teaspoonful Q.I.D.

MEDICINAL PROPERTIES

Diuretic
Renal Tonic
Diaphoretic
Alterative

COMBINATIONS:

For scurvy	Equal Parts:	
Blood diseases	Burdock	
Bronchitis	Yellow Dock	Standard Infusion
Skin diseases	Sarsaparilla	

PLANT IDENTIFICATION #19

ARNICA
Leopard's Bane

ARNICA ALPINA
Arnica fulgens
Arnica cordifolia

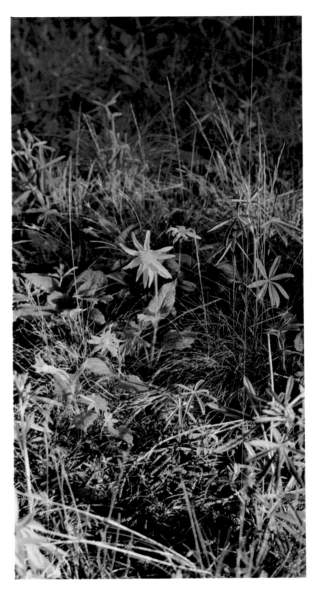

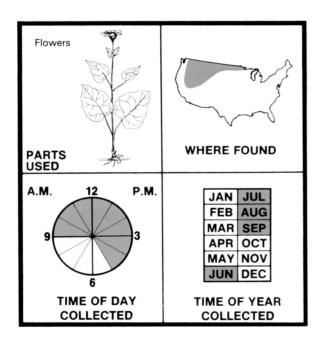

Flowers **PARTS USED**	**WHERE FOUND**
A.M. 12 P.M. 9 · 3 6 **TIME OF DAY COLLECTED**	JAN / JUL FEB / AUG MAR / SEP APR / OCT MAY / NOV JUN / DEC **TIME OF YEAR COLLECTED**

MEDICINAL USES:

- Bruises
- Swelling Associated with Sprains

- Bruises
- Swelling Associated with Sprains

PLANT INFORMATION:

Arnica is a member of the Sunflower Family (Compositae). This important plant is widely used by the Natural Healing Practitioners.

Arnica alpina, formerly called *Arnica montana,* is the main plant used, but several other species are effective. As the names suggest, it grows in high elevations and northerly latitudes.

Since its active principle is very potent, its uses should be directed closely by a practicing physician.

Several western species of Arnica have the ability to set viable seed without being fertilized. *Arnica alpina* has that characteristic.

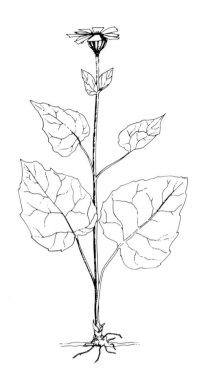

PREPARATION:

FOMENTATION (Special Preparation)

Pour boiling water over flowering head. Remove excess water and apply hot to the bruised or sprained area. Leave on until it is cold.

Repeat only 2 or 3 times.

EMERGENCY/Field Preparation

Pour boiling water over flowering heads. Remove excess water and apply hot to the bruised or sprained area. Remove when it has cooled down.

Repeat only 2 or 3 times.

MEDICINAL PROPERTIES
Counterirritant

PLANT IDENTIFICATION #20

GOLDEN SEAL

Orange Root, Yellow Root
Ground Raspberry, Tumeric Root
Indian Dye, Indian Tumeric

HYDRASTIS CANADENSIS

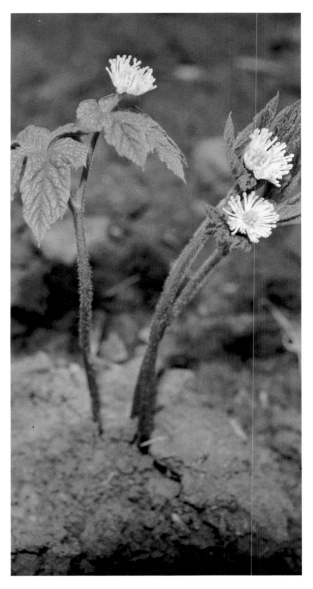

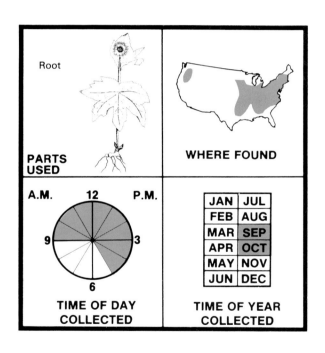

PARTS USED (Root)	WHERE FOUND
A.M. 12 P.M. 9 — 3 6 TIME OF DAY COLLECTED	JAN JUL / FEB AUG / MAR **SEP** / APR **OCT** / MAY NOV / JUN DEC TIME OF YEAR COLLECTED

MEDICINAL USES:

- All Mucous Membranes Inflammations and Dysfunctions
- Vaginitis
- Cankers
- Pyorrhea (Apply with tooth brush)

- Inflammed Uterus and Ovaries
- Gastritis
- Duodenitis
- Infant diarrhea
- Passive capillary bleeding
- Metrorrhagia

- Leucorrhea
- Menorrhagia
- Dyspepsia

- Cuts
- Wounds
- Sores

72

PLANT INFORMATION:

Golden Seal is in the Buttercup Family (Ranunculaceae) and has a wide variety of beneficial uses. Because of the great demand, it is now widely cultivated, and home cultivation is encouraged. It is native to the Eastern U.S., but is also found growing wild in Western Oregon and Washington.

It can be used singularily or in combination with many kinds of medicinal plants yielding extremely beneficial results.

Its use on a continual basis is discouraged, but should be taken not more than 7 to 10 days with 30 to 40 day intervals following each use period.

In its powdered form, it can be taken along on outings, hikes, and field trips as an emergency medication. For cuts or wounds, apply the powdered root directly over the injured area and cover with large leaved plants such as burdock (Arctium), Mules Ear (Wyethia), or Balsamroot leaves (Balsamorrhiza). Common lettuce or cabbage leaves may also be used. Wrap and cover to hold in place.

When drying the root, the optimum temperature is 80°F and to prevent rot or mildew, drying must be complete. This can be determined by feeling the sliced roots. If they feel cool, drying is not complete.

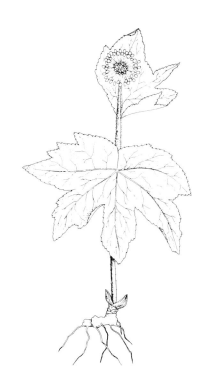

PREPARATION:

TINCTURE (See Section 6 for General Tincture Preparation Information)

STANDARD TINCTURE

1 part green root by weight, 2 parts 60% alcohol

Dosage: 1 to 4 drahms T.I.D.

POWDERS (See Section 8 for General Powder Preparation Information)

STANDARD POWDERED CAPSULE
10 to 40 Grains

Dosage: 1 capsule once or twice daily.

EMERGENCY/Field Use

Use described in Plant Information Section

DECOCTION (See Section 7 for General Decoction Preparation Information)

Boil 1 oz. chopped and contused root in ½ pint water for 3 minutes.

Dosage: 1 fluid ounce 4 to 6 times daily.

MEDICINAL PROPERTIES
Tonic
Alterative
Astringent
Antiperiodic
Antiseptic

COMBINATIONS:

For Extreme Nervousness { ¼ oz. of Powdered: Lady Slipper Golden Seal Lobelia Cayenne } Mix in 1 cup of warm water Dose: as needed

POULTICE PREPARATION

DEFINITION: Poultices are soft, moist plant tissue applied warm or hot to the surface area of the body to alleviate pain, or to draw out inflammations and infections. The plant may be mixed with other plants or other poultice making materials.

PROCEDURE

STEP 1.

Pour one cup bruised herb (linseed meal, etc.) into 2 ½ cups of boiling water.

STEP 2.

Stir constantly to uniform texture.

STEP 3.

Pour hot paste onto a prepared flannel cloth. Spread evenly. Fold to form an elongated bag.

STEP 4.

Apply as hot as can comfortably be withstood. Cover with hot water bottle to keep hot for as long as possible.

STEP 5.

Have a second poultice ready to apply as soon as the first becomes cold.

GENERAL INSTRUCTION CONCERNING POULTICES

- The best poultices are made from ground or granulated herbs.
- The area to be covered by a poultice may need to be washed with hydrogen peroxide.
- The main object of applying poultices is to have the warmth and moisture retained as long as possible.
- Do not re-warm a poultice once used.
- When using herbs in a powdered form, mix just enough water to make a thick paste. Paste should be about one inch thick.
- When using granulated herbs, mix with hot water, cornmeal, or some other meal to make a thick paste.
- If green leaves are used, mash, beat, or contuse the plant. Steep in hot water for a couple of minutes and apply to affected area.
- Apply hot, but not so as to burn the skin surface.
- In some cases, the plant juices will stain clothing and may need to be covered with a piece of plastic.

SEVERAL OLDTIME POULTICE RECIPES

1. BREAD POULTICE

Heat bread crumbs with fresh whole milk. Stir to thickness desired. Add a small amount of lard to prevent the skin from becoming wrinkled.

Use: (Infections)

2. RASPBERRY LEAF POULTICE

Make a strong infusion with the leaves. Add this to crumbled crackers and powdered Slippery Elm bark. Put in a touch of ginger and stir to poultice texture.

Use: (Rubefacient)

3. CARROT POULTICE

Shred four ounces of carrot - add one ounce of corn meal. Add enough boiling water to make poultice texture. Onion may replace carrot for Onion poultice.

Use: (Inflammation and Suppurations)

4. CAYENNE PEPPER POULTICE

Add equal parts of Cayenne Powder and Slippery Elm. Infuse warm water to form a poultice.

Use: (Counterirritant)

5. MUSTARD POULTICE

Mix two or three fluid ounces of boiling water with 2½ ounces of ground Mustard. Now separately mix 6 to 8 fluid ounces of boiling water with 2½ ounces of ground linseeds.

Now mix the two separate mixtures together to form a poultice.

Use: (Rubefacient)

6. LINSEED OR FLAXSEED POULTICE

Mix 10 fluid ounces of boiling water to 4½ ounces of Linseed meal. Stir to poultice consistency.

Use: (Emollient-Drawing)

7. GENERAL HEALING POULTICE

Combine 12 parts of Bayberry root bark with 6 parts of ginger powder and 1 part each of cayenne powder and cloves. To this add 20 parts of Slippery Elm powder. Mix in hot water to poultice texture. Add small amount of lard.

Use: (Stimulant - Astringent)

8. SPICE POULTICE

This poultice is prepared from ordinary household spices - namely Mustard, Ginger, Cinnamon, and Allspice in equal parts. Add a warm vinegar to form poultice.

Use: (Aromatic - Anodyne)

9. POTATO POULTICE

Shred raw potato into fine granules. Close the eye and apply without heating. Hold in place with gauze patch and secure with cloth retainer.

Use: (Pink-eye Inflammation)

FIELD NOTES/LABORATORY NOTES

Section V

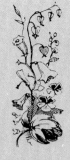

Lobelia

The Intelligent Plant

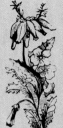

Black Cohosh

The Hormone Balancer

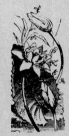

Raspberry

The Pre-birth Herb

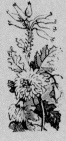

Squaw Vine

Indian Medicine Herbal

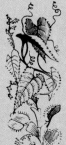

Scullcap

The Nerve Control Herb

PLANT IDENTIFICATION #21

LOBELIA
Indian Tobacco

LOBELIA INFLATA
Lobelia purpurascens
Lobelia species

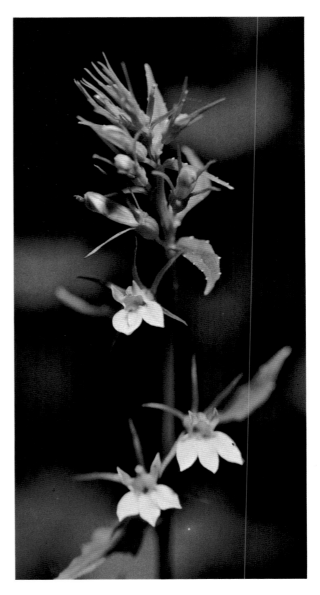

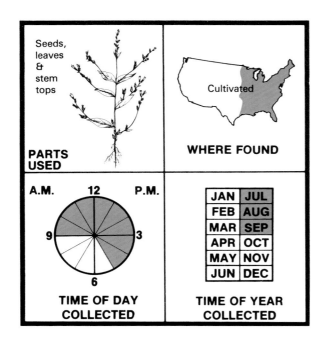

PARTS USED Seeds, leaves & stem tops	**WHERE FOUND** Cultivated
TIME OF DAY COLLECTED A.M. 12 P.M.	**TIME OF YEAR COLLECTED**

JAN	**JUL**
FEB	**AUG**
MAR	**SEP**
APR	OCT
MAY	NOV
JUN	DEC

MEDICINAL USES:

- Coughs
- Bronchitis
- Whooping Cough
- Pneumonia
- Convulsions

- Croup
- Asthma
- Earache
- Tetanus
- Ringworm

- Pneumonia (external compress or plaster)
- Boils
- Painful skin infections

PLANT INFORMATION:

This marvelous healing herb is in the Bellflower Family (Campanulaceae). It is one that should be kept on hand either as a stored, dried botanical or as an ornamental house plant.

The tender flowering tops and seeds are the most important part of the plant to be used, but the leaves are also medicinal.

Medicinal preparation can be in several forms; e.g., powders, poultices, fluid extract, tinctures, infusions and syrups.

Care should be taken to regulate the dosage to the age given.

It is an excellent pulmonary expectorant and strong results can be expected and should be prepared for.

Always give a stimulant herb before, during, or after the administration of this plant.

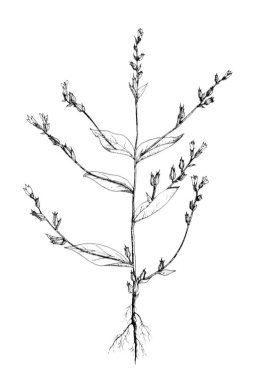

PREPARATION:

INFUSION (See Section 7 for General Infusion Preparation Information)

STANDARD INFUSION

Dosage: ½ to 1 wineglassful B.I.D. for 2 or 3 days

TINCTURE (See Section 6 for General Tincture Preparation Information)

See Special Tincture Combinations Page 191.

POULTICE (See Section 4 for General Poultice Preparation Information)

STANDARD POULTICE

Apply as hot as possible as needed.

MEDICINAL PROPERTIES

Expectorant
Emetic
Antispasmodic
Diuretic
Nervine
Diaphoretic

A. 5 Week Pre-parturition Herbal Medicant.
(Medication to ease labor and delivery)
Start with 2 oz. each of the powdered plants:

COMBINATIONS:

B. Lobelia
Black Cohosh
Raspberry Leaves
Penny Royal
Squaw Vine
Blessed Thistle

C. Incapsulate in .05 gelatine capsules. Take 1 each day for 31 days.

79

PLANT IDENTIFICATION #22

BLACK COHOSH

Black Snake Root, Bugwort
Bugbane, Squaw Root
Rattleweed, Rich Weed, Macrotnys

CIMICIFUGA RACEMOSA

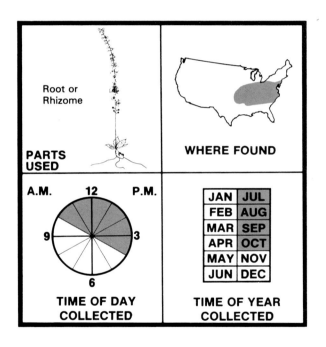

PARTS USED	WHERE FOUND
Root or Rhizome	

TIME OF DAY COLLECTED

A.M.	12	P.M.
9		3
	6	

TIME OF YEAR COLLECTED

JAN	JUL
FEB	AUG
MAR	SEP
APR	OCT
MAY	NOV
JUN	DEC

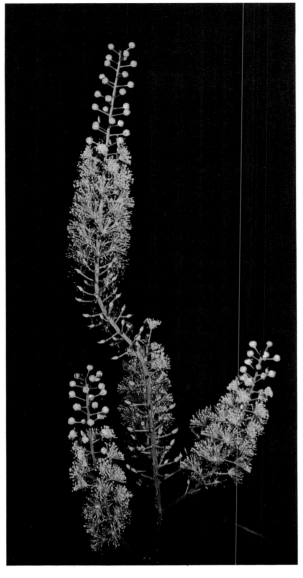

MEDICINAL USES:

- Chorea
- Epilepsy
- High Blood Pressure
- D.T.s
- Asthma
- Insect bites (wash)

- Pleurisy
- Endocarditis
- Pericarditis
- Intercostal neuralgia
- Rheumatic Pains
- Insures proper third stage in *partus preparatus*

- Whooping Cough
- D.T.s.
- Relieves stomach pain associated with flatulent colic.
- Tones organs of secretion in the stomach.
- Tones peristaltic actions of the digestive system.

PLANT INFORMATION:

Black Cohosh is an Eastern plant in the Buttercup Family (Ranunculaceae).

Credit is given to the native Americans for knowledge of its uses and medicinal virtues.

It is used primarily for treating functional female disorders associated with menstration and parturition.

Many herbal practitioners consider Black Cohosh an equal to Digitalis in therapeutic action, but much safer to use.

One of its actions is to keep the body hormones in proper balance.

Black Cohosh is one of the five plants used in the Special 5 Week Herb Formula. (See Lobelia Preparation page 79).

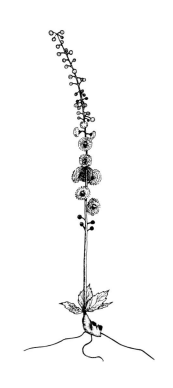

PREPARATION:

INFUSION (See Section 7 for General Infusion Preparation Information)

STANDARD INFUSION

Dosage: 3 to 5 drahms T.I.D.

TINCTURE (See Section 6 for General Tincture Preparation Information)

Use one part (by weight) root to 10 parts (by weight) Alcohol. Macerate 14 days. Strain, bottle and cork.

Dosage: 1 to 20 minims T.I.D.

SYRUP (Special Preparation)

Boil 3 ounces of the cut herb in simple syrup or karo syrup. Dilute with water until it becomes the right consistency. Strain through a double cheesecloth, bottle and cork.

Dosage: 1 tablespoonful every 4 hours.

MEDICINAL PROPERTIES

Emmenogogue	Astringent
Alterative	Tonic
Anthirheumatic	Sedative
Nervine	Expectorant

PLANT IDENTIFICATION #23

RASPBERRY
Western Black Raspberry
Western Red Raspberry
Red Raspberry

RUBUS STRIGOSIS
Rubus idaeus L.
Rubus leucodermis
Rubus villosus

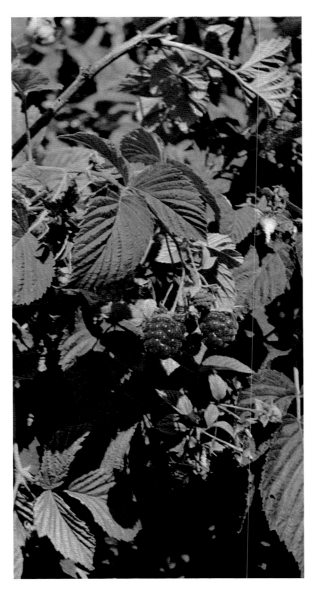

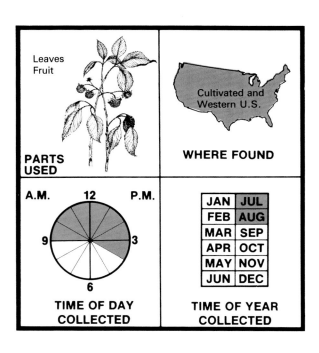

Leaves Fruit **PARTS USED**	Cultivated and Western U.S. **WHERE FOUND**
A.M. 12 P.M. 9 3 6 **TIME OF DAY COLLECTED**	JAN / JUL FEB / AUG MAR / SEP APR / OCT MAY / NOV JUN / DEC **TIME OF YEAR COLLECTED**

MEDICINAL USES:

- Cankers & Mouth and Throat Sores (as a Gargle)
- Dysentary & Diarrhea (especially in children)
- Increases milk supply
- Ophthalmia (as a wash)
- Leucorrhea (as an injection

PLANT INFORMATION:

Raspberry is a member of the Rose Family (Rosaceae). This is one of the most readily available plants for therapeutic use and should be collected and dried for use during the winter and spring months.

During the latter time of gestation, the expectant mother should substitute their regular tea (if they drink tea) with raspberry leaf tea. The result would be less instrument birth and practically no hemorrhaging after parturition.

It is one of the five plants used in the Special Five Week Herb Formula which eases labor and delivery discomforts. (See page 79)

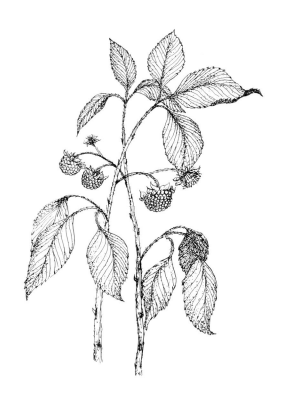

PREPARATION:

INFUSION (See Section 7 for General Infusion Preparation Information)

STANDARD INFUSION

Drink Freely

COMBINATIONS:
For Constipation:
1 oz. Raspberry Leaves
1½ oz. Flax Seeds

STANDARD
INFUSION
Standard Infusion

MEDICINAL PROPERTIES

Astringent
Stimulant
Parturient

PLANT IDENTIFICATION #24

SQUAW VINE
Partridge Berry
One-Berry
Checkerberry
Winter Clover
Deerberry

MITCHELLA REPENS

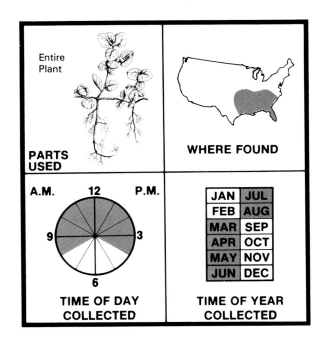

Entire Plant

PARTS USED

WHERE FOUND

A.M.   12   P.M.

9   3

6

TIME OF DAY COLLECTED

JAN	JUL
FEB	AUG
MAR	SEP
APR	OCT
MAY	NOV
JUN	DEC

TIME OF YEAR COLLECTED

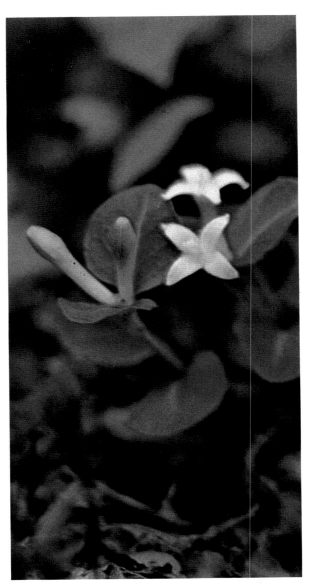

MEDICINAL USES:

- Proper embryo and Fetal Development
- Promotes proper Lactation Development
- Relieves:
  Menorrhagia
  Amenorrhea
  Dysmenorrhea
- Dysentary (especially during pregnancy)

- Treatment of Sore nipples due to nursing

PLANT INFORMATION:

Mitchella is in the Madder Family (Rubiaceae) and a near relative of Teasel, Elderberry and Honeysuckle.

This plant should be used during the entire nursing period for those mothers breastfeeding their babies.

It helps regulate the menstrual cycle after the new baby is several months old and in many cases is superior to hormone therapy.

Squaw Vine is one of the five plants used in the special 5 week herbal formula which eases labor and delivery discomforts. (See page 79 combinations).

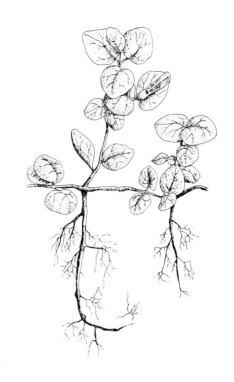

PREPARATION:

INFUSION (See Section 7 for General Infusion Preparation Information)

Mix 1 teaspoonful of Powdered plant in one cup of boiling water.

Dosage: 2 or 3 cups per day.

OINTMENT (See Section 5 for General Ointment Preparation Information)

(1) Make strong infusion of berries. Bathe nipples. Then add small amount of olive oil or cream to portions of infusion.

(2) Infuse berries to a strong tea. Add ¼ oz. tincture of myrrh and 1 oz. of glycerine.

Dosage: Apply frequently

MEDICINAL PROPERTIES
Diuretic
Astringent
Tonic
Alterative
Parturient

COMBINATIONS:

Ointment { Mix the juices of Partridge Berry and the juices of Hawksbeard with 2 oz. of glycerine. } For Sore Nipples

PLANT IDENTIFICATION #25

SCULL CAP
Madweed
Quaker Bonnet
Hood Wort

SCUTELLARIA LATERIFLORA

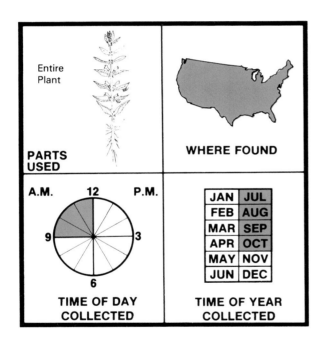

Entire Plant **PARTS USED**	**WHERE FOUND**
A.M. 12 P.M. 9 3 6 **TIME OF DAY COLLECTED**	JAN / JUL FEB / AUG MAR / SEP APR / OCT MAY / NOV JUN / DEC **TIME OF YEAR COLLECTED**

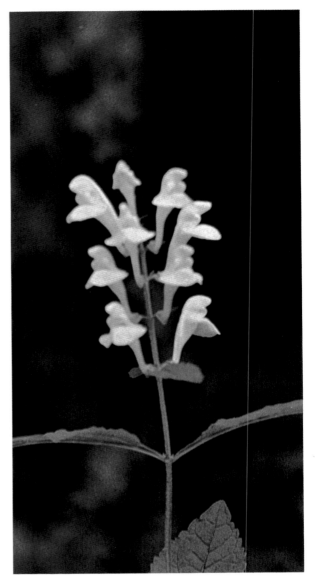

MEDICINAL USES:

- Chorea
- Nerve Tonic
- Insomnia
- D.T.'s
- Hydrophobia
- Convulsions

- Chorea
- Nerve Tonic
- Insomnia
- D.T.'s
- Hydrophobia
- Convulsions

PLANT INFORMATION:

Scull Cap is in the Mint Family (Labiatae). It is fairly widespread in the U.S. and can be collected without much difficulty.

As with all the mints, care must be taken to insure proper collecting and drying techniques. Always store in a moisture-proof airtight container to prevent the plant from absorbing water from the atmosphere.

Do not store for more than one year. The potency levels drop rapidly after that amount of time has passed. It can then be transformed into a tincture to preserve the plant's efficiency.

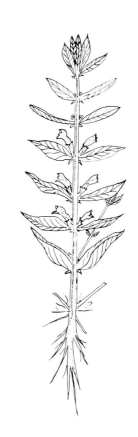

PREPARATION:

INFUSION (See Section 7 for General Infusion Preparation Information)

STANDARD INFUSION

Dosage: ½ teacup as frequently as needed. Usually about 4 times each day.

TINCTURE (See Section 6 for General Tincture Preparation Information)

One part by weight mashed plant to 5 parts (45%) Alcohol. Steep 8 days. Strain, bottle and cork.

Dosage: 1 to 30 minims T.I.D.

MEDICINAL PROPERTIES

Tonic
Nervine
Antispasmodic
Astringent

OINTMENT PREPARATION

DEFINITION: Ointments are semi-solid preparations for external application. They are derived from animal or vegetable oils and also from petroleum bases with other supplemental substances added to make them more usable.

Modern bases are available which make excellent ointment preparations.* Various non-commerical ointment substances can be obtained in your own locality without much difficulty.

OINTMENT BASES:

1. Lanolin (Wool Fat)
2. Goose Grease
3. Lard
4. Olive Oil
5. Sesame Seed Oil
6. Cotton Seed Oil
7. Hydrogenated Vegetable Oil
8. Peanut Oil
9. Safflower Oil
10. Mineral Oil
11. Petrolatum (Petroleum Jelly)
12. Glycerin

To give the above ointment bases firmness Bee's Wax (White or Yellow) and Parafin wax are supplemental additives. The amount of these hardeners added depends upon how climatically hot it is during the summer.

Equipment needed to compound usable Ointment.

Porcelain mortar
and pestle.

Plate Glass

Balanced handle
spatula.

Bunsen burner

88

*See R.B.C. p. 16

OINTMENT PREPARATION

METHODS OF GETTING MEDICINAL PLANT SUBSTANCES INTO THE OINTMENT BASE.

Method I. Preparation by Incorporation.

STEP ONE

Reduce the medicaments into a fine powder (see page 130.)

STEP TWO

Select Ointment Base for your particular purpose.*

STEP THREE

Use a small portion of bases to be used. Gradually incorporate the powder to form a smooth nucleus. Continue to add base to obtain right texture and consistency.

Method II. Preparation by Fusion.

STEP ONE

Prepare a water bath (using a double boiler-type pan) to melt the fusion ingredients. For example, bees wax, parafin, lanolin. Start melting the materials with the greatest fusion temperatures and add those materials with lower melting points.

STEP TWO

Remove from heat (a safe distance away from heat source) and slowly add fine, powdered herb.

STEP THREE

Stir constantly while adding medicament.

STEP FOUR   (Optional)

If necessary, strain to remove unwanted material. Use clean, fine-weaved cloth.

STEP FIVE

Stir until preparation is homogenous and cooled to a uniform, thick ointment.

*Depending upon your application, the following classifications are made:

(1) Non-penetrating Ointment - used for epidermal therapy. It is needed especially where an emollient - protective is indicated.
    Example: petrolatum, waxes or combination of both.

(2) Deep-penetrating Ointment - used to penetrate into the deep layers of the skin. They are indicated when inflammation is present.
    Example: vegetable oils, lard, lanolin or combination of these.

FIELD NOTES/LABORATORY NOTES

Section VI

Five Botanicals
Tincture and
Fluid Extract Preparation

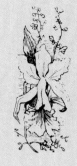

Yellow Dock

The Iron King

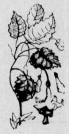

Bearberry

The Kidney Toner

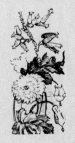

Gravel Root

The Gravel Expeller

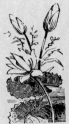

Chickweed

The Cosmopolitan Herb

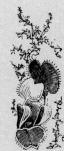

Camomile

The Powerful "Little Apple"

PLANT IDENTIFICATION #26

YELLOW DOCK
Sour Dock, Bitter Dock
The Dock, Curly Dock

RUMEX CRISPUS
Rumex obtusifolia

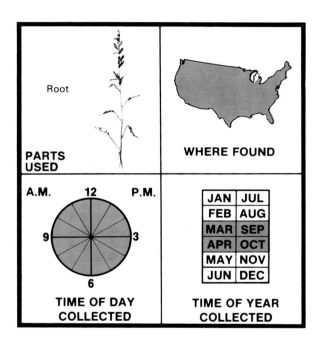

Root **PARTS USED**	**WHERE FOUND**
A.M. 12 P.M. 9 3 6 **TIME OF DAY COLLECTED**	JAN JUL / FEB AUG / MAR SEP / APR OCT / MAY NOV / JUN DEC **TIME OF YEAR COLLECTED**

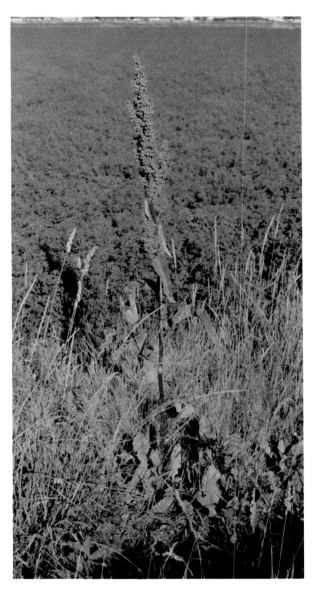

MEDICINAL USES:

- Blood Purifyers
- Skin eruptions
- Scorbutic diseases
- Scrofula
- Iron anemia
- Thyroid Dysfunction

- Skin eruptions
- Itch
- Piles

PLANT INFORMATION:

Yellow dock is in the Buckwheat Family (Polygoneaceae). The root contains the medicinal substance, and should be collected when these substances are concentrated in the root system in the spring or late fall.

It should be cut or sliced and dried for future use.

The young leaves can be cooked as a pot herb and constitutes a good source of natural Vitamin C.

It has one of the richest supplies of assimilable organic iron found in nature. It is prepared by boiling ½ pound of the crushed root in 1 pint of sugar water for five minutes. This forms a syrup which helps its ingestion. Strain and bottle for future use.

Caution: Avoid drinking commercial coffee or tea while taking yellow dock for these substances are incompatible.

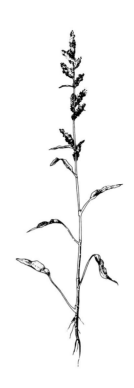

PREPARATION:

DECOCTION (See Section 7 for General Decoction preparation)

STANDARD DECOCTION

Dosage: 1 tablespoonful in cup of water T.I.D.

OINTMENT (See Section 5 for General Ointment preparation)

Boil 1 ounce of sliced root in brown vinegar for 20 minutes. Blend softened root pulp with white vaseline. Add ½ teaspoon (level) of U.S.P. sulphur. Mix well.

Dosage: Apply topically to skin surface as needed.

MEDICINAL PROPERTIES

Alterative
Laxative
Tonic
Astringent
Detergent
Antiscorbutic

PLANT IDENTIFICATION #27

BEARBERRY

Bears' Grape, Uva Ursi
Upland Cranberry, Rockberry
Mountain Box, Trailing Arbutus

ARCTOSTAPHYLOS UVA-URSI L.
Arctostaphylos species

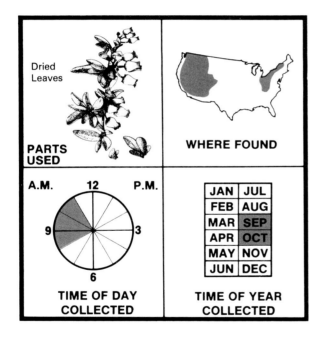

Dried Leaves

PARTS USED

WHERE FOUND

A.M.   12   P.M.

9   3

6

TIME OF DAY COLLECTED

JAN	JUL
FEB	AUG
MAR	SEP
APR	OCT
MAY	NOV
JUN	DEC

TIME OF YEAR COLLECTED

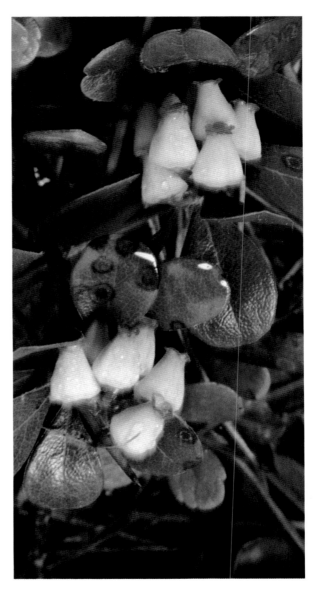

MEDICINAL USES:

- Diabetes
- Bladder and Kidney inflammation
- Atonic leucorrhea
- Urethritis
- Prostatic hypertrophy

- Diabetes
- Bladder and Kidney inflammations
- Atonic leucorrhea
- Urethritis
- Prostatic hypertrophy

PLANT INFORMATION:

Bearberry is in the Heath Family (Ericaceae). The leaves are collected in the fall of the year, and only those fully freen colored leaves should be selected for use.

They should be dried in single layers at temperatures between 70° and 100°F. and turned at regular intervals. Do not use direct sunlight in the drying process as this will bleach the leaves rendering them less potent.

After the drying is complete, place them in an airtight container since they are hygroscopic and will absorb moisture from the air.

Both scientific names refer to its common name Bearberry. *Arcto* = Bear + *staphylos,* cluster of grapes (Greek) and *Uva* = grape + *Ursi* = Bear (Latin)

This plant grows at elevations above 6000 feet and is found growing abundantly close to mountain roads.

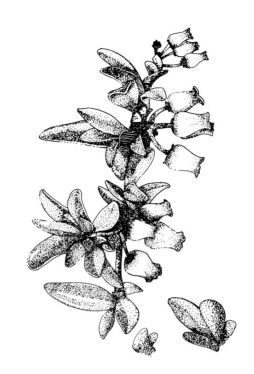

PREPARATION:

INFUSION (See Section 7 for General Infusion preparation)

STANDARD INFUSION

Dosage: One wine glass full T.I.D.

COMBINATIONS:

Antiseptic effect on the Urinary mucous membrane

Equal parts

Bearberry ½ ounce
Poplar bark ½ ounce
Marshmellow root ½ ounce

STANDARD INFUSION

Wineglassful doses T.I.D.

For Diabetes
Equal parts

Bearberry leaves
Blueberry leaves

STANDARD TINCTURE
(Prepare as the tincture above)

20 drops T.I.D.

TINCTURE (See Section 6 for General Tincture preparation)

STANDARD TINCTURE

(A good brandy can be used as a menstruum)

Dosage: 10 to 20 drops in water T.I.D. or Q.I.D.

MEDICINAL PROPERTIES

Astringent
Diuretic
Renal Sedative & Antiseptic
Carminative
Tonic

PLANT IDENTIFICATION #28

GRAVEL ROOT
Joepye-weed, Queen of the Meadow

EUPATORIUM PURPUREUM
Eupatorium perfoliatum

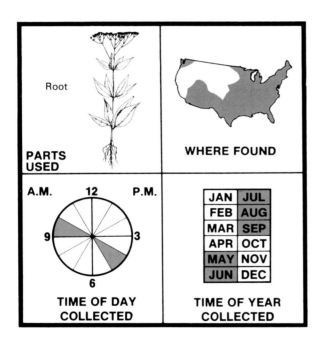

PARTS USED — Root

WHERE FOUND

TIME OF DAY COLLECTED — A.M. / P.M.

TIME OF YEAR COLLECTED

JAN	JUL
FEB	AUG
MAR	SEP
APR	OCT
MAY	NOV
JUN	DEC

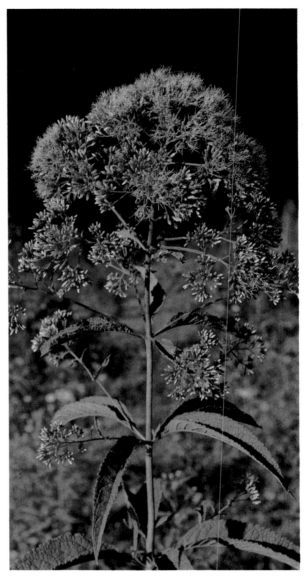

MEDICINAL USES:

- Rheumatism
- Neuralgia of the Lower Back
- Gravel in the Gall Bladder, Kidney, and Urinary Bladder
- Dropsy
- Urethritis
- Prostatis

- Rheumatism
- Neuralgia of the Lower Back
- Gravel in the Gall Bladder, Kidney, and Urinary Bladder
- Dropsy
- Urethritis
- Prostatis

- Rheumatism
- Neuralgia of the Lower Back
- Gravel in the Gall Bladder, Kidney, and Urinary Bladder
- Dropsy
- Urethritis
- Prostatis

PLANT INFORMATION:

Gravel Root is a member of the Sunflower Family (Compositae), and as the name suggests it's use is to prevent or treat gall stones, urinary bladder stones, and kidney stones.

It is an effective plant in treating kidney and bladder atonies which are associated with painful urination (dysuria), and bloody urine (hematuria).

There are two species which are medicinal. *Eupatorium purpureum,* the pink-flowered Gravel Root, and *Eupatorium perfoliatum,* called the White-flowered Boneset.

Early herbalists learned many of the medicinal uses of this plant from the Indians. It is primarily an Eastern plant, but is is now listed in several Western floras.

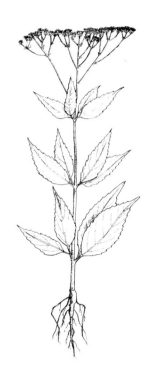

PREPARATION:

DECOCTION (See Section 7 for General Decoction preparation information)

STANDARD DECOCTION

Dosage: 1 to 3 Fluid ounces T.I.D.

TINCTURE (See Section 6 for General Tincture preparation information)

1 part Ground Root
Macerate in 5 parts 40% alcohol for 1 week.

Dosage: 1 tablespoonful B.I.D. or T.I.D.

POWDERED PLANT (See Section 8 for General Powdered plant preparation information)

Powder and place in 30 to 60 grain gelatine capsules.

Dosage: 1 Capsule T.I.D.

MEDICINAL PROPERTIES
Diuretic
Stimulant
Tonic
Astringent
Relaxant

PLANT IDENTIFICATION #29

CHICKWEED
Stitchwort, Scarwort, Satin Flower
Adder's mouth

STELLARIA MEDIA
Stellaria jamesiana
Stellaria longifolia
Stellaria longipes
Stellaria umbellata
Stellaria obtusa

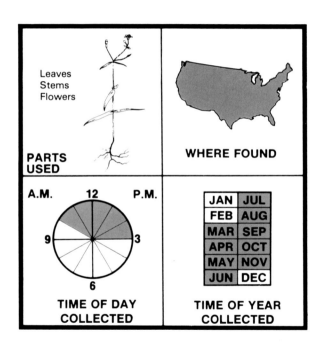

PARTS USED — Leaves, Stems, Flowers

WHERE FOUND

TIME OF DAY COLLECTED

TIME OF YEAR COLLECTED

JAN	JUL
FEB	AUG
MAR	SEP
APR	OCT
MAY	NOV
JUN	DEC

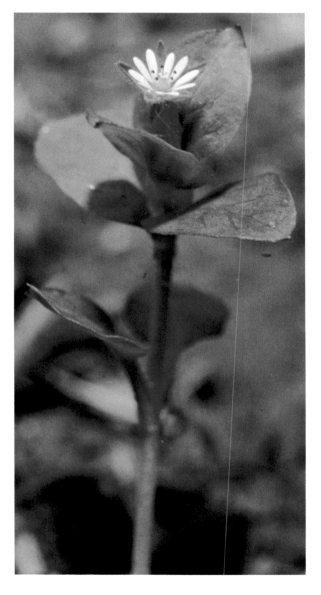

MEDICINAL USES:

- Carbuncles
- External Abscesses
- Boils
- Scalds

- Bronchitis
- Pleurisy
- Internal Inflammation
- Constipation

- Carbuncles
- Hemorrhiods
- External abscesses

98

PLANT INFORMATION:

Chickweed is in the Pink Family (Caryophyllaceae) and is the first cousin to the Carnation. It is one of the most widely distributed plants in the world, ranging from the equator to within the artic circle.

It is considered a garden pest, but this is a minor problem compared to its medicinal usefulness, and its use as a salad ingredient.

Chickweed is a good source of Vitamin C, and as the name implies, is relished by young chicken.

In the U.S. it is best collected from May to July.

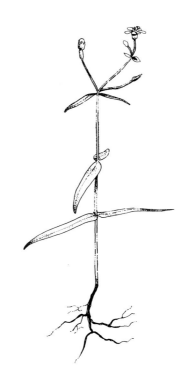

PREPARATION:

POULTICE (See Section 4 for General Poultice Preparation)

STANDARD POULTICE

(Fresh or Dried Leaves may be used)

Apply as needed

INFUSION (See Section 7 for General Infusion Preparation)

STANDARD INFUSION

Dosage: 1 wineglassful Q.I.D.

OINTMENT (See Section 5 for General Ointment Preparation)

Add 1 cup finely chopped plant to 1 pound boiling lard. Cool and strain through a clean, white, sterile cloth.

Use as needed.

MEDICINAL PROPERTIES

Demulcent
Emollient
Pectoral
Refrigerant
Alterative

PLANT IDENTIFICATION #30

CAMOMILE
Ground Apple
Manzanilla

ANTHEMIS NOBILIS

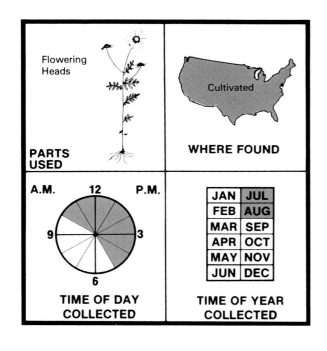

Flowering Heads

PARTS USED

Cultivated

WHERE FOUND

A.M. 12 P.M.

9 · 3

6

TIME OF DAY COLLECTED

JAN	JUL
FEB	AUG
MAR	SEP
APR	OCT
MAY	NOV
JUN	DEC

TIME OF YEAR COLLECTED

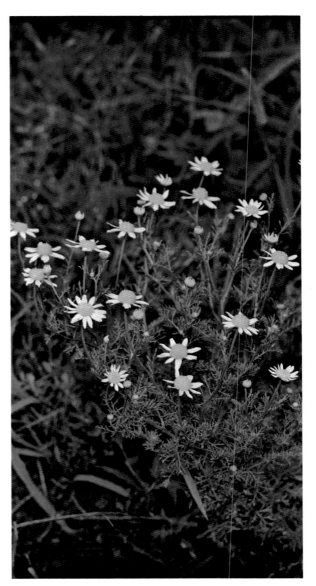

MEDICINAL USES:

- Flatulent Colic
- Colds
- Atonic dyspepsia
- Amenorrhea
- Dysmenorrhea

- Flatulent Colic
- Cradle Cap

PLANT INFORMATION:

Camomile is a member of the Sunflower Family (Compositae). It is a pleasant garden plant with an aromatic scent resembling the smell of an apple. The Spanish name of camomile is Manzanilla, meaning "a little apple".

The tea should always be prepared in a covered vessel to prevent the escape of the vapors.

Camomile has antiseptic properties and contains calcium and potassium.

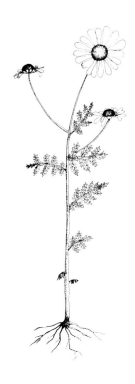

PREPARATION:

INFUSION (See Section 7 for General Infusion Preparation Information)

STANDARD INFUSION
Steep at least 10 minutes before straining.

Dosage: Drink freely as needed.

OIL OF CAMOMILE (Special Preparation)
Mix 40% alcohol (2½ fluid ounces) with mashed flowering heads. (3 oz.). Macerate in closed glass jar for 24 hours. Add 16 fluid ounces of pure olive oil. Heat for 12 hours at temperatures between 50 and 60 degrees centigrade. Strain and express into a sealable container.

Oil — for cradle cap use as needed.
For Colic — Dosage: 1 to 3 drops as needed.

MEDICINAL PROPERTIES
Tonic
Stomachic
Anodyne
Antispasmodic

TINCTURE PREPARATION

DEFINITION: Tinctures are preserved plant extracts produced by soaking a given amount of plant material (usually in powdered form) in direct proportion to an extracting solution (usually alcohol) called the menstruum. It is sometimes referred to as a dilute Fluid Extract.

STANDARD TINCTURE (Procedure A or B)

Ratio of Plant material to Menstruum. 1 gram to 10 ml.

1.5 ounces to 1 pint (English) } Workable
45 grams to 500 milliliters (Metric) } Quantities

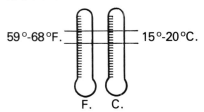

Ideal Maceration and Percolation temperatures

PROCEDURE A

MACERATION TECHNIQUE:

STEP 1.
Macerate (indicated amount) amount of plant material with proper amount of menstruum. Make sure bottle or container has a good sealing top.

STEP 2.
Let material soak for approximately 2 weeks at temperatures listed as ideal, above. Keep away from the direct sunlight.

STEP 3.
Shake bottle twice each day.

STEP 4.
Decant and filter extract. Pour off supernatant into a clean bottle. Where possible, express liquid from plant into bottle.

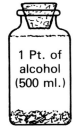

1 Pt. of alcohol (500 ml.)

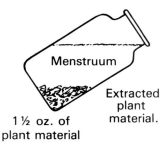

Menstruum

1 ½ oz. of plant material

Extracted plant material.

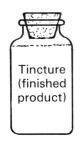

Tincture (finished product)

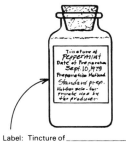

STEP 5.
Cork (or rubber stopper), label and store safely. Be sure to seal container tightly with an adequate sealing lid. Store in a safe place away from small children. Under lock and key if possible.

Label: Tincture of _____
Date of Preparation _____
Preparation Method _____
Not for Sale - for private use by producer only.

PROCEDURE B

PERCOLATION TECHNIQUE:

STEP 1.
Place desired amount of plant material (powdered or green) into a mixing jar.

STEP 2.
Add enough of given amount of uniformly moistened material.

STEP 3.
Macerate for twenty-four hours.

STEP 4.
Place moist plant material in a conical perculator. Pack firmly to where perculation is not slow or too rapid.

STEP 5.
Check rate of perculation. (see page 104).

STEP 6.
Add sufficient menstruum to perculate 500 milliliters (1 pint) in receiving jar.

1.5 ounces of plant material in soaking menstruum

STEP 7.
Cap bottle and label for storage and future use. (see step 5, Procedure A).

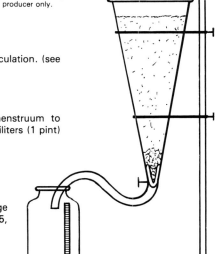

FLUID EXTRACT

DEFINITION: An alcohol preparation of a vegetable extract containing the active constituents in a definite ratio of plant material to solvent. It is sometimes called a 100% tincture.

STANDARD FLUID EXTRACT
Ratio of Plant Material to Menstruum —— 1 gram to 1 milliliter of Menstruum.

500 grams to 500 milliliter } Workable
1 pound of 1 pint. } Quantities

PROCEDURE A

STEP 1.
Macerate powdered or granulated plant material in appropriate menstruum.

STEP 2.
Soak for 10 days (or as specified). Keep away from direct sunlight and keep temperature at ideal range.

STEP 3.
Express (squeeze) through a clean cloth into a container. Filter into a bottle and cap or cork to seal. Label (see opposite page for labeling instructions).

PROCEDURE B

Follow steps 1 and 2 of Procedure A.

STEP 3.
Using a conical perculator, first place a filter paper in the lower "neck" of the apparatus. Sometimes a sterile rock or pebble is placed next to hold the filter paper in place. (depending on the nature of the perculate, a menstruum soaked piece of cotton can be placed in the neck of the perculator.)

STEP 4.
Pack moist plant material into the perculator. Pack firmly to where rate of perculation is at desired speed. If the amount of moistened plant material will adequately fit in the perculator, maceration can be done within the perculator. (Step 2)

STEP 5.
When perculation is to begin, add sufficient menstruum to perculate through the plant mass until the extracted fluid reaches the predetermined height in the calibrated receiving bottle. Two or three perculations can be accomplished with the original plant material before it is totally exhausted. (each extraction is of course less potent than the previous one.)

STEP 6.
Seal (cork or rubber stopper), label, and safely store.

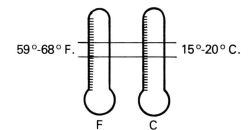

59°-68° F.   15°-20° C.

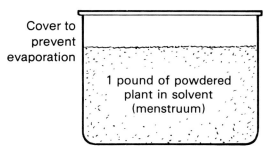

Cover to prevent evaporation

1 pound of powdered plant in solvent (menstruum)

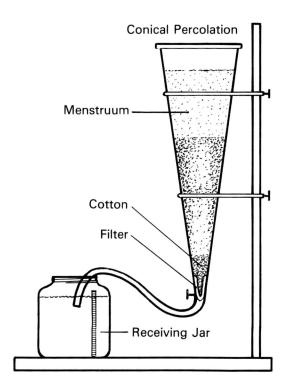

Conical Percolation

Menstruum

Cotton

Filter

Receiving Jar

Section VII

Five Botanicals
Infusion and
Decoction Preparation

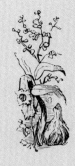

Blue Flag

The Shield Protector

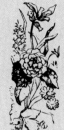

Lady Slipper

The Orchid's Contribution

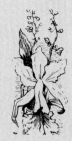

Couch Grass

The Dog Doctor

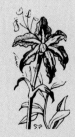

Yarrow

The Military Herb

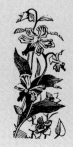

Dandelion

The Official Herb

PLANT IDENTIFICATION #31

BLUE FLAG
Water Flag, Flag Lily
Liver Lily, Iris

IRIS VERSICOLOR
Iris missouriensis
Iris virginica

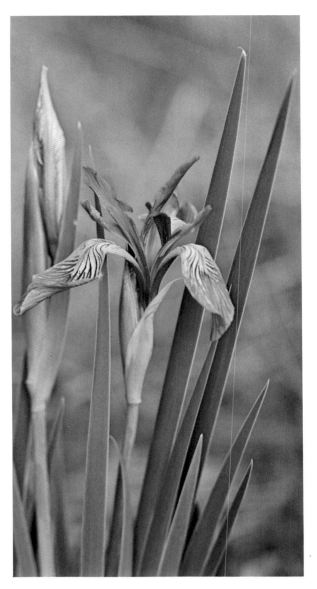

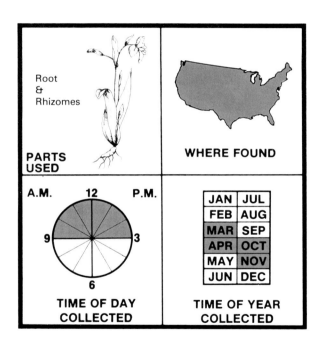

Root & Rhizomes

PARTS USED

WHERE FOUND

A.M. 12 P.M.
9 3
6

TIME OF DAY COLLECTED

JAN	JUL
FEB	AUG
MAR	SEP
APR	OCT
MAY	NOV
JUN	DEC

TIME OF YEAR COLLECTED

MEDICINAL USES:

- Inflammed fingernails and toenails
- Abscesses
- Suppurations
- Painful infections

- Swollen lymph and thyroid glands
- Excessive salivation
- Constipation

- Swollen lymph and thyroid glands
- Removes Catabolic wastes

PLANT INFORMATION:

Blue Flag is in the plant Family (Iridaceae) commonly called the Irises. Most species contain the same medicinal properties and can be used for the same purpose.

Its use as an emetic should be discouraged because of its harshness to the gastrointestinal system.

The roots have no specific odor, but the taste is acrid.

A principal use is in the treatment of enlarged thyroid and lymphatic glands (non-malignant)

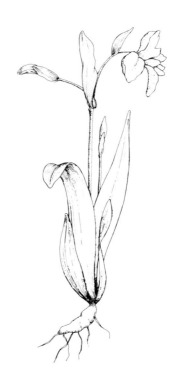

PREPARATION:

POULTICE (See Section 4 for General poultice preparation information)

Gather fresh roots in the spring or autumn. Chop and mash to a pulp. Apply hot to infected part. Cover to keep heat and moisture in. Apply as needed.

DECOCTION (See Section 7 for General decoction preparation information)

Add ½ ounce of dried root to one quart of boiling water. Boil for 3 minutes. Steep for 10 minutes. Cool and strain.

Dosage: 1 to 2 fluid ounces B.I.D.

TINCTURE (See Section 6 for General tincture preparation information)

Mix two parts of 50% alcohol to one part of the contused root. Pour into a well stoppered bottle and macerate for 8 days. Decant, strain and filter extracted liquid.

Dosage: 5 to 30 minims T.I.D.

COMBINATIONS:

Equal parts of Blue Flag and Purple Cone Flower. Add 2 parts by weight 50% alcohol.

Removal of Catabolic wastes
STANDARD TINCTURE

**MEDICINAL
PROPERTIES**
Choleretic
Alterative
Anodyne

PLANT IDENTIFICATION #32

LADY SLIPPER

Nerve Root, Yellow Lady Slipper
American Valerian, Yellow Noah's
Ark, Yellow Umbil

CYPRIPEDIUM PUBESCENS
Cypripedium luteum
Cypripedium parviflorum

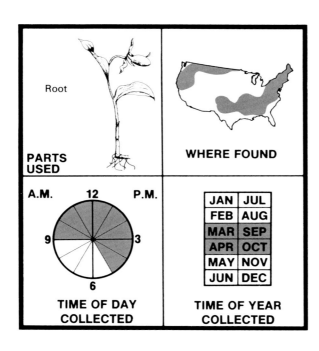

Root

PARTS USED

WHERE FOUND

A.M. 12 P.M.

9   3

6

TIME OF DAY COLLECTED

JAN	JUL
FEB	AUG
MAR	SEP
APR	OCT
MAY	NOV
JUN	DEC

TIME OF YEAR COLLECTED

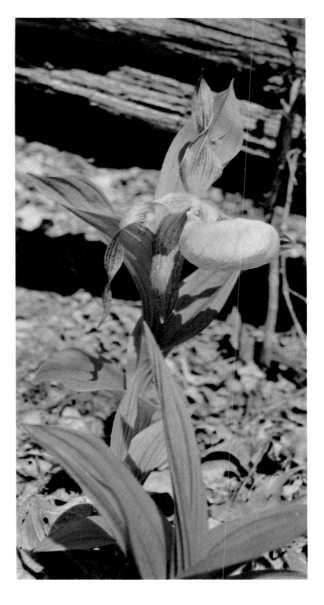

MEDICINAL USES:

- Loss of strength or energy
- Insomnia
- Female Climacteric
- Facilitates parturition

- Loss of strength or energy
- Insomnia

- Pelvic Neuralgia
- Insomnia

- Mental and Emotional upsets

PLANT INFORMATION:

Lady Slipper is the only plant in the Orchid Family (Orchidaceae) used medicinally in the U.S.

It can and should be cultivated to preserve the genus from the strong impact of collection.

All species of this genus are effective.

Its therapeutic value and action simulates that of the plant Valerian, being without poisonous or narcotic effects.

Overdoses can lead to mental depressions.

It principally grows in the eastern U.S. and its early medicinal uses were learned from the Indians.

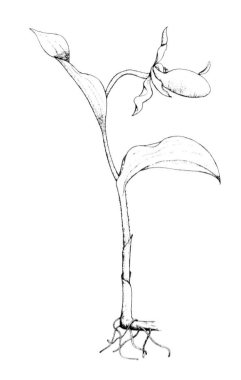

PREPARATION:

INFUSION (See Section 7 for General Infusion Preparation Information)

1 Dram dried root to 4 ounces of boiling water. Steep 10 minutes.

Dosage: 4 to 8 fluid ounces daily

TINCTURE (See Section 6 for General Tincture Preparation Information)

Add one part (by weight) of mashed root to 2 parts (by weight) of 40% alcohol. Let stand for 8 days in cool place. Strain, bottle and seal.

Dosage: 5 to 20 minims T.I.D.

FLUID EXTRACT (See Section 6 for General Fluid Extract Preparation Information)

Add one part (by weight) of mashed root to one part (by weight) of 40% alcohol. Let stand 8 days in cool place. Strain, bottle and seal.

Dosage: 5 to 20 minims T.I.D.

POWDERED PLANT (See Section 8 for General Powdering Preparation Information)

Grind to a fine powder and capsulate.

Dosage: 30 to 60 grains T.I.D.

MEDICINAL PROPERTIES

Nervine
Stimulant
Antispasmodic
Sedative

PLANT IDENTIFICATION #33

COUCH GRASS
Dog Grass
Quitch
Quick Grass
Crab Grass

AGROPYRON REPENS

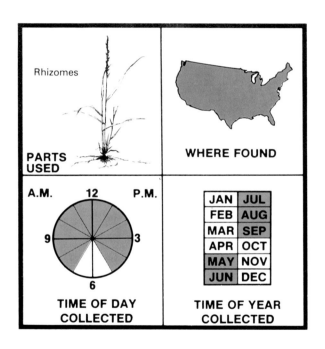

Rhizomes

PARTS USED

WHERE FOUND

A.M.   12   P.M.

9   3

6

TIME OF DAY COLLECTED

JAN	JUL
FEB	AUG
MAR	SEP
APR	OCT
MAY	NOV
JUN	DEC

TIME OF YEAR COLLECTED

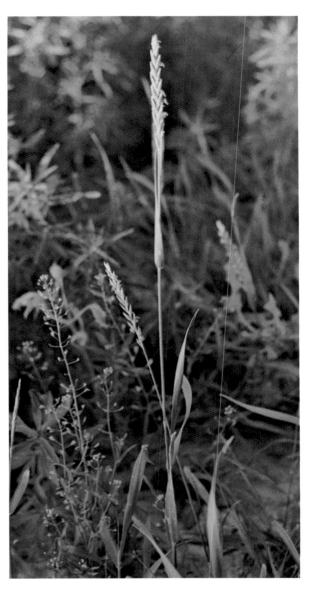

MEDICINAL USES:

- Painful or difficult urination

- Tonic to the Renal (Kidney) Structures

110

PLANT INFORMATION:

This is one of the few plants found in the Grass Family (Gramineae) which is considered medicinal. It is well known to gardeners who know it as a terrific lawn pest.

It reproduces both by seed and by vegatative underground stems called rhizomes. It is these brown rhizomes which are collected for medicinal use.

Dogs chew it frequently, which accounts for it being commonly called Dog Grass.

In the West it is best known as Crab Grass.

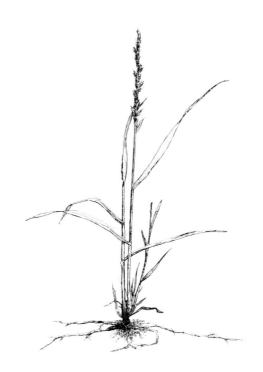

PREPARATION:

INFUSION (See Section 7 for General Infusion Preparation Information)

STANDARD INFUSION

1 ounce of chopped rhizomes steeped in one pint of boiling water for 20 minutes.

Dosage: One wineglassful T.I.D.

MEDICINAL PROPERTIES

Aperient
Demulcent
Diuretic

PLANT IDENTIFICATION #34

YARROW

Gordoloba, Nosebleed, Soldiers
Milfoil, Thousand leaf, Green arrow
Woundwort, Carpenter's grass
Sanguinary, Old man's pepper
Dog daisy, Berbe Militaris

ACHILLEA MILLEFOLIUM L.
Achillea lanulosa
Achillea sp.

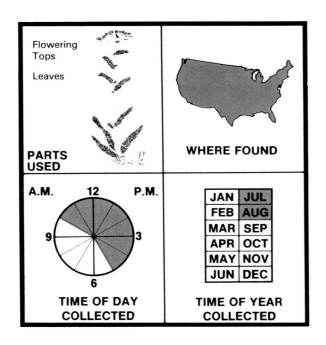

Flowering Tops

Leaves

PARTS USED

WHERE FOUND

A.M. 12 P.M.

9   3

6

TIME OF DAY COLLECTED

JAN	JUL
FEB	AUG
MAR	SEP
APR	OCT
MAY	NOV
JUN	DEC

TIME OF YEAR COLLECTED

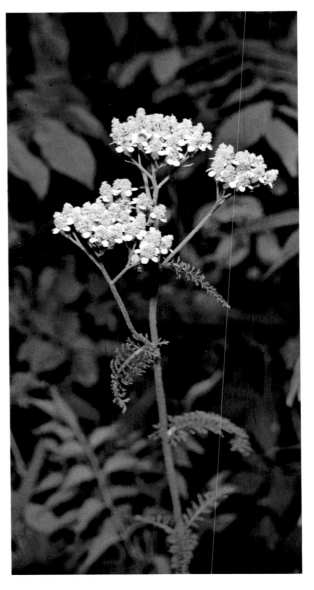

MEDICINAL USES:

- Colds and Flu
- Fever
- Hemorrhage
- Pulmonary and Alimentary Canal Catarrah
- Excessive Menses

- Cuts
- Wounds
- Piles

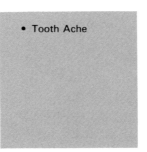

- Tooth Ache

- Colds and Flu
- Fever
- Hemorrhage
- Pulmonary and Alimentary Canal Catarrah
- Excessive Menses

PLANT INFORMATION:

Achillea is a member of the Sunflower Family (Compositae). For many centuries this plant has been used as a *vulnernary,* hence the common names: soldier's wound wort, or Berbe Militaris, the Military Herb. Brigham Young, the Mormon Prophet said of this plant: Fortunate is the person who knows how to use yarrow in the last days.

Achillea is the *generic* name of this plant, so named because legend says that Achilles used the plant to stop the bleeding wounds of his soldiers. It is most commonly called Yarrow and is found growing along roadsides, on hillsides, and low mountain ranges. It can also be cultivated.

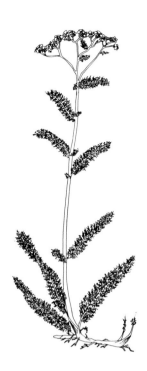

PREPARATION:

INFUSION (See Section 7 for General Infusion Preparation Information)
STANDARD INFUSION
One ounce chopped leaves steeped in one pint of boiling water for 20 minutes.
Dosage: One wineglassful T.I.D.

EMERGENCY/Field Use:
Remove several leaves—Chew to a pulpy poultice. Pack around tooth that is aching.

OINTMENT (See Section 5 for General Ointment Preparation Information)
Gather ten ounces of the fresh leaves and flowering tops. Contuse to a pulp. Add to 20 ounces of melted Lard. Carefully heat over a direct flame until all of the moisture has evaporated. Strain through clean linen cloth into a container.
Apply liberally to Cuts, Wounds or Piles.

TINCTURE (See Section 6 for General Tincture Preparation Information)
Gather the whole herb when the flowers are in full bloom. Contuse to a pulp. Add equal part of 40% alcohol. Allow to stand for 8 days in a cool, dark place. Filter, bottle and cork.
Dosage: 5 to 25 minims T.I.D.

MEDICINAL PROPERTIES
Tonic, Stimulant
Emmenagogue
Diaphoretic
Astringent

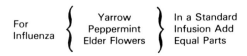

For Influenza { Yarrow Peppermint Elder Flowers } In a Standard Infusion Add Equal Parts

PLANT IDENTIFICATION #35

DANDELION

Cankerwort
Lion's tooth
Puff ball
Priest Crown

TARAXACUM OFFICINALE

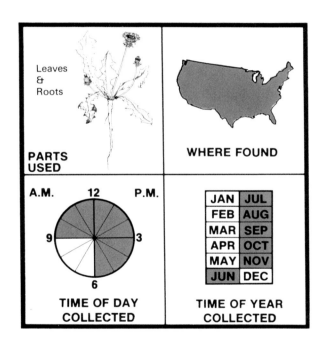

PARTS USED	WHERE FOUND
Leaves & Roots	

TIME OF DAY COLLECTED	TIME OF YEAR COLLECTED

JAN	JUL
FEB	AUG
MAR	SEP
APR	OCT
MAY	NOV
JUN	DEC

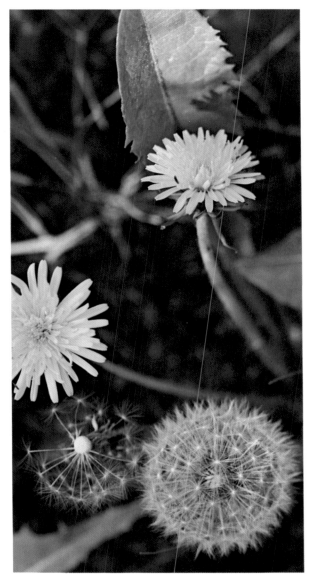

MEDICINAL USES:

- Liver and Kidney Disorders
- Dyspepsia
- Stomach Tonic
- Gout
- Rheumatism
- Dermatitis

- Liver and Kidney Disorders
- Dyspepsia
- Stomach Tonic
- Gout
- Rheumatism
- Dermatitis

PLANT INFORMATION:

Dandelion is a neglected (and hated) useful plant. The dried and chopped roots should be used in place of the more harmful coffees and teas.

A tasty brew can be made by roasting equal parts of dandelion, dried acorn, and barley.

This plant is very nutritive and has therapeutic value in treating liver and kidney disorders.

The species name is officinale, referring to its former-day medicinal use. It was an official plant remedy of the Roman Government.

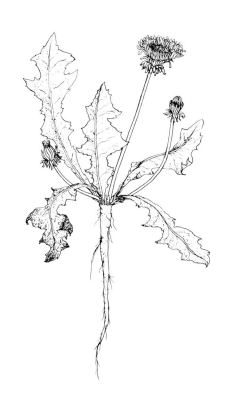

PREPARATION:

INFUSION (See Section 7 for General Infusion Preparation Information)

Pour boiling water over 1 cup of leaves. Steep for 35 minutes. Strain and drink cold. Sweeten to taste with honey.

Dosage: As desired

POWDERED PLANT (See Section 8 for General Powdering Preparation Information)

Place one teaspoonful of powdered root in one cup of boiling water. Steep for 35 minutes. Drink when cold.

Dosage: Three cupfuls daily

MEDICINAL PROPERTIES

Hepatic
Tonic
Stomachic
Aperient

COMBINATIONS:

Tonic { Dandelion Golden Seal } Standard Infusion

INFUSION PREPARATION

DEFINITION: Infusions are aqueous solutions of plant extracts prepared at a temperature just below the boiling point. The plant material may be dried or moist. Like Decoctions, infusions are temporary extracts, and unused portions should be discarded after several hours. An infusion is commonly called a "Tea".

STANDARD INFUSION

50 grams (coarsely comminuted) plant material in 1000 cc of distilled water
Workable Ratio: 1½ ounces of plant to 1 quart of water.

PROCEDURE A

STEP 1.

Place ground plant into a suitable glass or stainless steel container.

STEP 2.

Pour in just enough cold water to moisten plant material.

STEP 3.

Bring distilled water to a boil and pour over moistened plant material.

STEP 4.

Let steep for 15 minutes, then pass product through a strainer.

PROCEDURE B

STEP 1.

Place 1½ ounces of leaves, flowers, and/or stems into a suitable container. Add 1 quart of cold water.

STEP 2.

Add heat. When water begins to boil, remove from heat and let cool for 5 minutes or until it cools to drinkable temperature.

STEP 3.

Strain and express juices through a strainer into a quart jar.

STEP 4.

Add enough water to fill quart capacity.

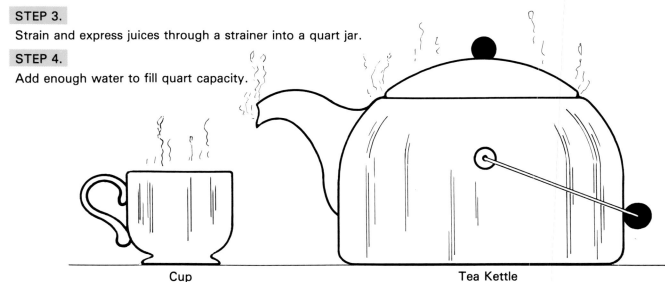

Cup   Tea Kettle

DECOCTION PREPARATION

DEFINITION: Decoctions are aqueous solutions of plant extracts prepared at a boiling temperature. They differ from Infusions generally in that roots and other course plant structures make up the decoction substances. This is a temporary extract and should not be kept over 5 or 6 hours. Make fresh preparation as needed.

STANDARD DECOCTION

50 grams (generally of coarsely comminuted) plant material in 1000 cc of cold water.
Workable Ratio: 1½ ounces of plant to 1 quart of water.

PROCEDURE

STEP 1.

Place ground plant into a suitable vessel provided with a cover (lid). Never use aluminum or iron cookware. Porcelain or heat-resistant glassware is preferred.

STEP 2.

Pour in one quart (1000 cc) of cold water. Mix to uniformity.

STEP 3

Place container over heat. Once material comes to a boil, set timer for 15 minutes of boiling time.

STEP 4.

Remove from heat and cool to about 100° F.

STEP 5.

Pour decoction through a strainer, expressing juices from the plant material. You should have slightly less than the 1000 cc, so pour additional cold water over the "marc" through the strainer and into the holding vessel until the 1 quart level is reached.

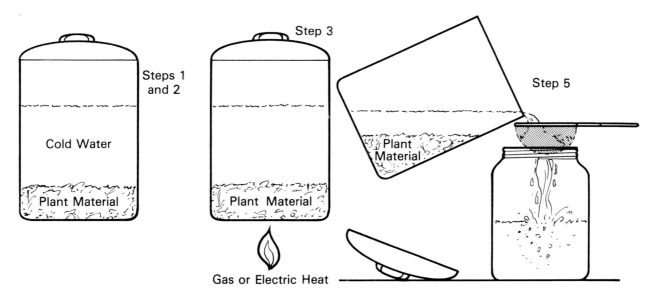

117

FIELD NOTES/LABORATORY NOTES

Section VIII

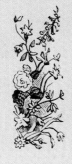

Linum

The Master Poultice Herb

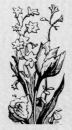

Elderberry

The Multi-purpose Herb

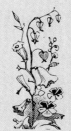

Willow

The Natural Pain Reliever

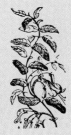

Blue Cohosh

The Pappose Root

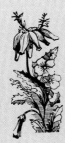

Brighams Tea

The Pioneer Herb

PLANT IDENTIFICATION #36

LINUM
Flaxseed, Poultice Seed

LINUM USITATISSIMUM
Linum lewisii

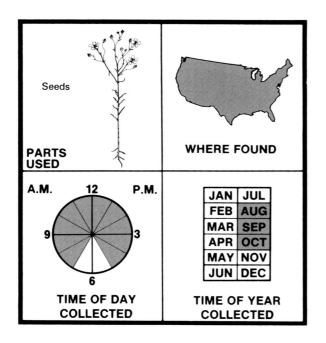

Seeds

PARTS USED

WHERE FOUND

A.M. 12 P.M.
9 3
6

TIME OF DAY COLLECTED

JAN	JUL
FEB	AUG
MAR	SEP
APR	OCT
MAY	NOV
JUN	DEC

TIME OF YEAR COLLECTED

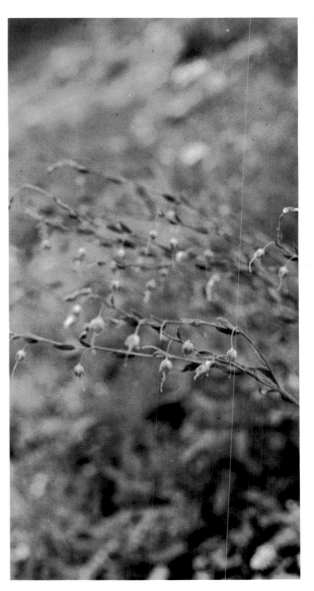

MEDICINAL USES:

- Inflammations of:
  Lungs
  Bronchi
  Thyroid
  Abdomen

- Old Sores
- Boils
- Carbuncles
- Tumors
- Infections

- Coughs
- Asthma
- Pleurisy

PLANT INFORMATION:

Linum is in the Flax Family (Linacaea). Two main species are present in the United States, *Linum lewisii,* discovered by the famous Captain Merriweather Lewis, and *Linum usitatissimum,* the flax of commerce (from which the fine linen is produced) and a Native of the Black Sea area.

The mature and cured seeds of this plant make an excellent poultice. The seeds are rich in flax oil (about 40% by weight) and the seed coat is high in mucilage.

Flaxseed poultices are excellent for drawing out body toxins, and for reducing body inflammations.

Depending upon its intended use, other ground plants such as Comfrey, Mullein, Mustard, and Lobelia seeds can be blended with Linum to enhance its healing qualities.

Always use the seeds before the milling and refining process has removed the oil content.

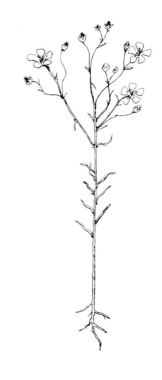

PREPARATION:

POULTICE (See Section 4 for General Poultice preparation)

- Collect ¼ ounce of matured Flaxseeds.
- Grind to a fine powder.
- Add fine powder to 1 pint of boiling water. Mix while adding to prevent lumps.

Apply as needed.

INFUSION: (See Section 7 for General Infusion Preparation Information)

STANDARD INFUSION

Dosage: In wineglass doses. T.I.D.

MEDICINAL PROPERTIES

Pectoral
Demulcent
Emollient

PLANT IDENTIFICATION #37

ELDERBERRY

American Elder
Pipe Tree
Bore Tree
Bour Tree

SAMBUCUS CANADENSIS L.
Sambucus nigra L.

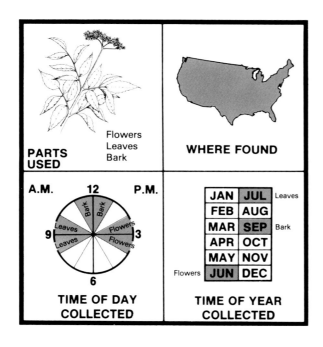

PARTS USED — Flowers, Leaves, Bark

WHERE FOUND

TIME OF DAY COLLECTED
A.M. 12 P.M.
Bark, Bark
Leaves, Flowers
Leaves, Flowers
9 — 3
6

TIME OF YEAR COLLECTED

JAN	JUL	Leaves
FEB	AUG	
MAR	SEP	Bark
APR	OCT	
MAY	NOV	
JUN	DEC	

Flowers

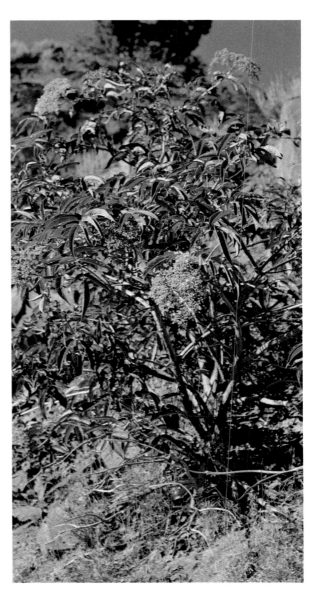

MEDICINAL USES:

- Weeping Eczema (Leaves)
- Rhus Poisoning (Leaves)
- Promotes Desquamation (Leaves)
- Cardiac Dropsy (Bark)
- Renal Dropsy (Bark)
- Wash for Inflamed Eyes (Flowers)

- Chilblains
- Bruises
- Sprains
- Indolent Skin Ulcers

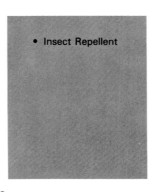

- Insect Repellent

122

PLANT INFORMATION:

Elderberry, or Elder, is a member of the Honeysuckle Family (Caprifoliaceae). It is a "first cousin" to snowberry (Symphocarpos) and the fragrant honeysuckle or twinberry (Lonicera).

The roots of Sambucus should not be used for they contain a toxic principle.

The leaves can be bruised and worn in a hat band, or under the hat to repel dipterous insects. (see emergency/field preparation below).

The bark from young trees collected in the autumn, makes a strong purgative, and in smaller doses is helpful in treating Cardiac and Renal Dropsy.

The flowers can be collected and mixed with pancake mix to enhance its flavor and texture.

Elderberry jam is an excellent source of Vitamin B_{17}.

A warm infusion of the flowers make a good wash for inflamed eyes.

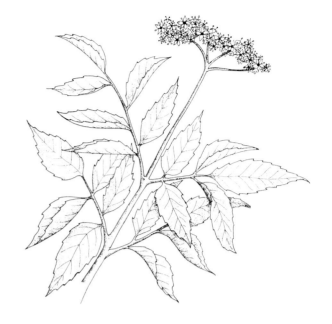

PREPARATION:

INFUSION (See Section 7 for General Infusion Preparation Information)

STANDARD INFUSION

Dosage: Taken hot or cold, Wineglassful Q.I.D.

EMERGENCY/Field Use

Mash leaves and rub on face.

or

Place bruised leaves under hat

or

Steep bruised leaves in olive oil for 7 days.

OINTMENT (See Section 5 for General Ointment Preparation Information)
Green Elder Ointment:
3 ounces of Elder leaves, 4 ounces Lard, 2 ounces prepared suet.
Add leaves to melted lard and suet. Heat until green color is extracted. Cool. Strain, place in jar.
Ointment of Flowers:
1 ounce of flowers, 3 ounces of hydrogenized codfish oil.
Heat for 20 minutes. Cool. Strain, place in jar.

MEDICINAL PROPERTIES
Stimulant
Carminative
Alterative
Disphoretic
Diuretic

PLANT IDENTIFICATION #38

WILLOW
Weeping Willow, Pussy Willow
Sandbar Willow, Black Willow

SALIX BABYLONICA
Salix discolor   Salix nigra
Salix exugia   Salix species

POPLAR
Cottonwood, Aspen

Populus tremuloides
Populus alba

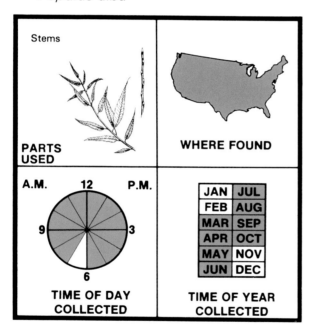

Stems **PARTS USED**	**WHERE FOUND**
A.M. 12 P.M. 9 3 6 **TIME OF DAY COLLECTED**	JAN JUL FEB AUG MAR SEP APR OCT MAY NOV JUN DEC **TIME OF YEAR COLLECTED**

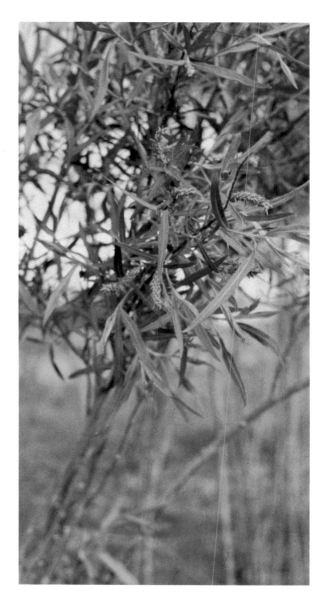

MEDICINAL USES:

- Headache
- Fever (Including Intermittent Fever)
- Psychic & Spastic Dysuria
- Vaginitis (Douche)
- Cuts, Bruises, Scratches (Antiseptic)
- Pain in Inflamed Joints, Muscles and Nerves.

- Malarial Periodicity
- Leucorrhea
- Fever and Headache

124

PLANT INFORMATION:

The Willows and Poplars belong to the same family (Salicaceae). All contain salicylic acid, but the willows are generally easier to work with in obtaining the active principle.

A pocket knife can be used to strip the bark from the stems (see illustration below). Cut between 15 to 20 1 inch strips to the cambium layer and remove from the plant. Add these strips "green" or dried to one pint of boiling water to make a decoction.

It is the salicylic content derived from the willows and poplars which relieve fever and headache pain.

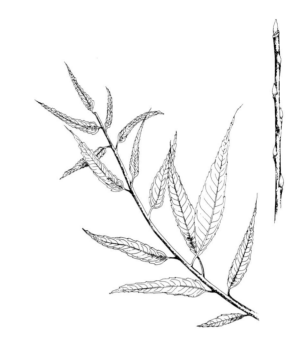

PREPARATION:

DECOCTION (See Section 7 for General Decoction Preparation Information)
1 ounce of green bark to 1 pint water.
STANDARD DECOCTION
Dosage: 2 fluid ounces T.I.D.

TINCTURE (See Section 6 for General Tincture Preparation Information)
STANDARD TINCTURE
Dosage: 10 to 30 minims T.I.D.

MEDICINAL PROPERTIES
Anodyne, Antiseptic
Astringent
Febrifuge, Tonic

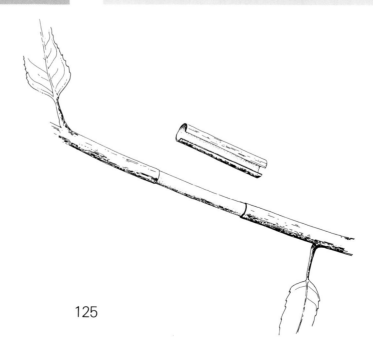

PLANT IDENTIFICATION #39

BLUE COHOSH
Sqaw Root, Pappoose Root

CAULOPHYLLUM THALICTROIDES

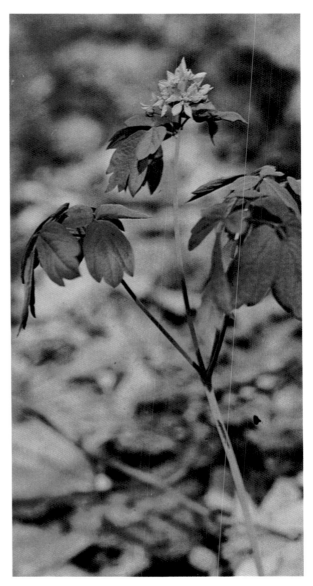

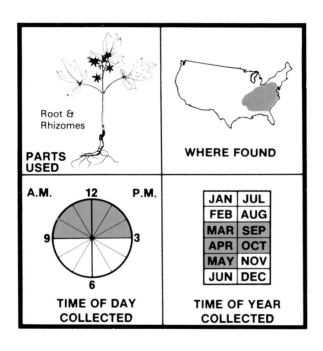

Root & Rhizomes **PARTS USED**	**WHERE FOUND**
A.M. 12 **P.M.** 9 — 3 6 **TIME OF DAY COLLECTED**	JAN JUL / FEB AUG / MAR SEP / APR OCT / MAY NOV / JUN DEC **TIME OF YEAR COLLECTED**

MEDICINAL USES:

- Partus preparatus
- Ovary pains
- Uterine subinvolution
- Vaginitis
- Leucorrhea
- Amenorrhea
- Dysmenorrhea

- Rheumatic conditions
- Neuralgia
- Relaxes Cramps and Spasms
- Metritis
- High Blood Pressure
- Palpitation of the Heart

126

PLANT INFORMATION:

Pappoose Root is a member of the Barberry Family (Berberidaceae). It is an Eastern plant and one used with great effect.

The Indian "Medicine Man" used this plant to treat female disorders associated with the labor and birth processes. It is an excellent uterine tonic.

It aids in the dilation of the cervix.

It should be used several weeks before and several weeks after parturition to insure normal uterine functioning.

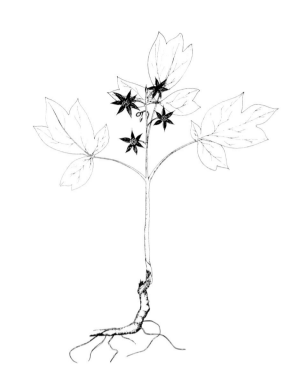

PREPARATION:

INFUSION (See Section 7 for General Infusion Preparation Information)

STANDARD INFUSION

Dosage: 4 drams every 3 hours.

FLUID EXTRACT (See Section 6 for General Tincture Preparation Information)

STANDARD FLUID EXTRACT

Dosage: 8 minums every 4 hours.

MEDICINAL PROPERTIES

Antispasmodic
Parturient
Diaphoretic
Emmenagogue
Uterine Tonic

PLANT IDENTIFICATION #40

BRIGHAM TEA
Miners' Tea, Mexican tea
Ephedra

EPHEDRA VIRIDIS
Ephedra nevadenses

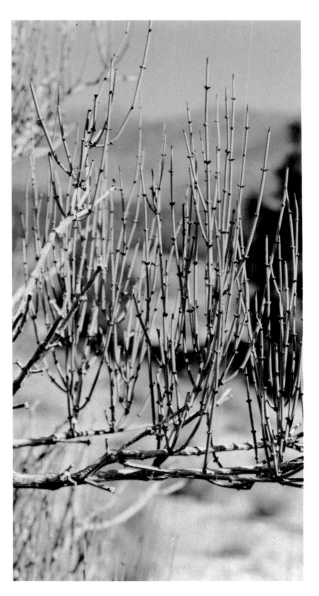

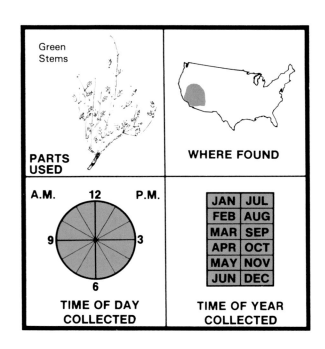

Green Stems		WHERE FOUND
PARTS USED		

TIME OF DAY COLLECTED	TIME OF YEAR COLLECTED

JAN	JUL
FEB	AUG
MAR	SEP
APR	OCT
MAY	NOV
JUN	DEC

A.M. 12 P.M.
9   3
6

MEDICINAL USES:

- Tonic

- Stimulant

- Normalize Blood Pressure

128

PLANT INFORMATION:

This plant is in the Ephedra Family (Ephedraceae). Botanically it is considered one of the "living fossils" being akin to the Horsetails in primitiveness of plant structure and form.

It appears to be transexual in some plant species. During many flowering seasons it will put forth staminate flowers (male), and in other growing seasons it will flower in the pistillate form (female).

To help make your desert experience more enjoyable, brew a handful of the green branches in a gallon can of water. Boil for about 15 minutes. The water will turn a nice amber color. Add brown sugar or honey. Serve either hot or iced. This drink will add enchantment and satisfaction to your evening desert campfire time.

The Asian species of this plant contains the drug Ephedrine, a vaso-constrictor.

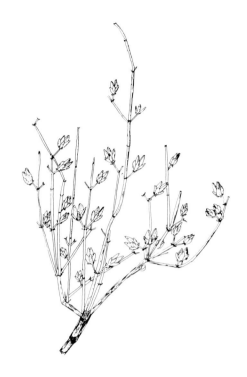

PREPARATION:

DECOCTION (See Section 7 for General Decoction Preparation Information)

STANDARD DECOCTION

(See Preparation Method in "plant information" Section above)

Dosage: Drink freely

MEDICINAL PROPERTIES
Stimulant
Tonic

POWDER PREPARATION

DEFINITION: Plants reduced in size to meet requirement for inclusion into capsules, ointments, and infusions, etc., is called powdering. This is accomplished by several methods listed on the opposite page.

GENERAL POWDERING INFORMATION:

(1) Select only good quality plant materials. They should be free from dirt, dust, and other adulterants. Brown or diseased plant parts should not be used.

(2) Powdering should be done just prior to the users actual need for the plants medicinal values. The active principles dissipates with the passage of time to about 12 to 15% per year. No powder should be kept over 4 years.

(3) Plant material should be extremely dry before the powdering process begins. Powdering is best accomplished with reduced environmental temperatures. (air conditioned area or during colder seasons.)

(4) Weight for weight, powdered plant is more potent than a herbaceous green plant. This is because the green plant has a high water content. To determine the ratio of green plant potency to dry plant strength, weigh the green plant before and after dessication. The weight difference will indicate the potency differences. For example, if one half of the weight is lost to drying, figure the green plant was 50% less potent than the same amount of the dried and powdered plant material.

(5) A problem with storing powdered botanicals is they must be stored so moisture and insects will not cause them harm. This problem can be solved by placing the dried plant in a clean paper bag and putting this bag in a sealable, plastic bag.

(6) Remember that fine powdered plants can be very flammable and should be kept away from open fire, or gas burners.

(7) When trying to reduce gummy or resinous plants to a powder, it may be necessary to add a little ether or high proof alcohol to the plant which allows it to be broken down into smaller particles without the sticky problems.

(8) Practice will greatly enhance your skill in using powdered plants. Since your work is for your own private use and not for sale or marketing, use only small amounts of the plant reserving your collected plant for future use.

POWDERING METHODS:

(A) Pre-reduction preparation of Plants.

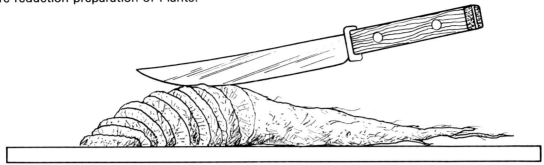

Some plant parts should be reduced in size while they are still green and freshly collected. Slicing and cutting to expose more surface area for drying can also serve to reduce the size of the plant for milling or grinding.*

Mills and plant grinders are available which are designed to reduce plant to granules or to fine powders*. Some are hand powered while others are electrically powered.

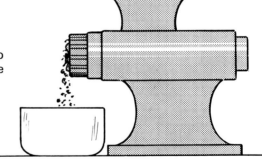

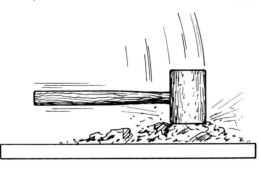

In many cases pulverizing with a hammer or mallet can reduce the dried plant to sizes where other powdering methods can be employed. Dried roots, coarse bark and thick stems can be comminuted by this technique.

(B) Fine reduction techniques.

After the plants have been reduced to a fairly small granular mass, or a more or less semi-coarse powder, a mortar and pestle can be used to further reduce the particle size.

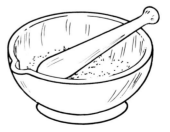

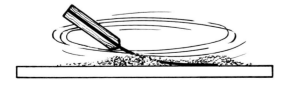

A spatula can be used to reduce particle size while incorporating medicaments into ointments and salves.

*See Milling Supply Sources (Page 12)

Section IX

Eight Botanicals
Techniques of
Plant Identification

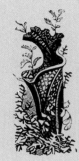

Aloe

The Ancient
Healing Wonder

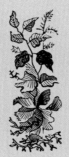

Bistorta

The Pearl of the
Marsh

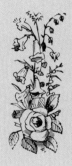

Purple Cone Flower

The Plant
of Venus

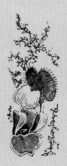

Potentilla

The "Little"
Potency Herb

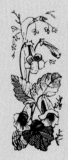

Gumweed

The Sticky
Physician

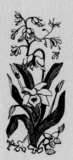

Chicory

The Refresher
Plant

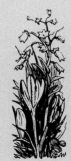

Yellow Clover

The Blood
Thinner Herb

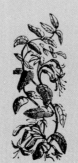

Cayenne

The Master
Stimulator

PLANT IDENTIFICATION #41

ALOE
> Aloes
> Turkey Aloes

ALOE VERA
> *Aloe socotrina*

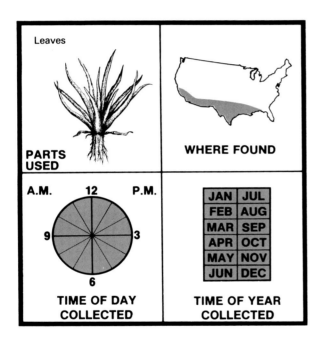

Leaves **PARTS USED**	**WHERE FOUND**
A.M. 12 P.M. 9 3 6 **TIME OF DAY COLLECTED**	JAN JUL FEB AUG MAR SEP APR OCT MAY NOV JUN DEC **TIME OF YEAR COLLECTED**

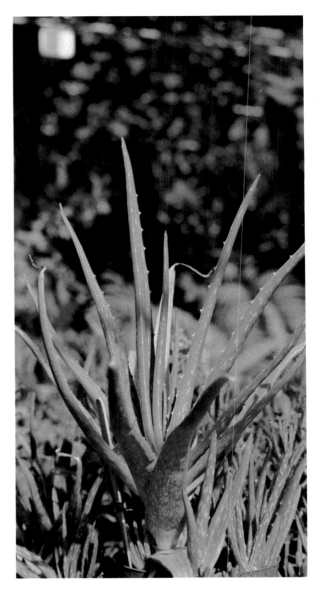

MEDICINAL USES:

- Internal body cleanser
- Antihistimine
- Relieves constipation
- Heals ulcers and stomach lesions.
- Antihelminthic (expels pinworms)

- Under-arm deodorant
- Acute burns
- Sunburns
- Removes scar tissue
- Hair conditioner
- Skin cuts and wounds

PLANT INFORMATION:

Aloe vera is a plant of the Lily Family (Liliaceae). Its natural habitat is in the warmer southern states.

It is a great therapeutic plant, but it should be used more to prevent body ailments and to maintain good body physiology.

It can be cultivated as an attractive house plant and will live the year round, making it very accessible to use.

The best juices come from plants three or four years old or older. It should be used fresh since special processes are required to ready it for storage.

This plant should be in every home.

It is one of the best natural under-arm deodorants available.

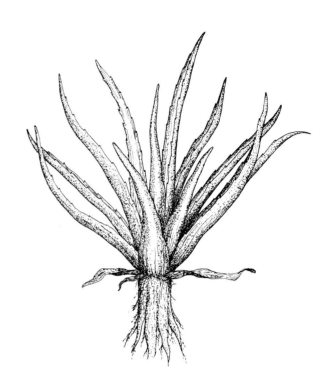

PREPARATION:

INFUSION (See Section 7 for General Infusion Preparation Information)

Cut leaf in cross section. Express light viscous juice from the leaf with your fingers into cold distilled water. 1 teaspoonful to the quart. Mix well. Make fresh after 48 hours. It will not keep.

Dosage: Two or three cupfuls daily.

OINTMENT (See Section 5 for General Ointment Preparation Information)

Aloe has a natural gel-type consistency. The expressed juices can be applied without further preparation.

PLANT IDENTIFICATION #42

PURPLE CONE FLOWER
Black Sampson
Narrow-leaf Coneflower

ECHINACEA ANGUSTIFOLIA
Echinacea purpurea

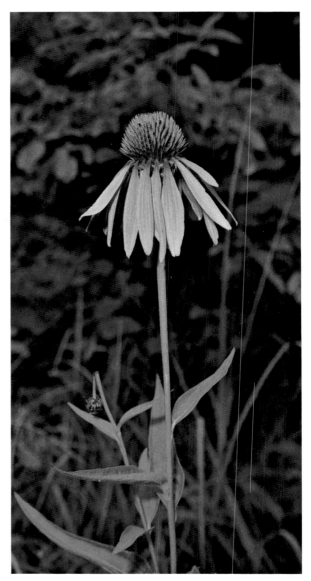

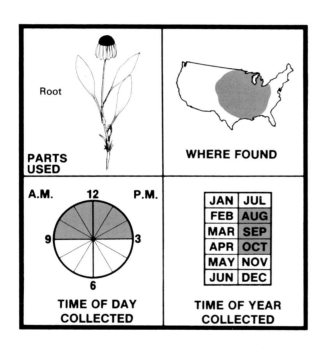

Root

PARTS USED

WHERE FOUND

A.M.   12   P.M.

9   3

6

TIME OF DAY COLLECTED

JAN	JUL
FEB	AUG
MAR	SEP
APR	OCT
MAY	NOV
JUN	DEC

TIME OF YEAR COLLECTED

MEDICINAL USES:

- Fermentative dyspepsia
- Blood Purifier for Boils, Carbuncles, Septicemia
- Tonsilitis and Sore Throat (as a gargle)
- Arthropod bites
  Scorpions
  Centipedes
  Spiders

- Fermentative dyspepsia
- Blood Purifier for Boils, Carbuncles, Septicemia
- Tonsilitis and Sore Throat
- Mouth Sores and Swollen Gums
- Arthropod bites

136

PLANT INFORMATION:

Coneflower is a member of the Sunflower Family (Compositae). It is one of the best blood purifiers with a wide spectrum of other uses.

The Eastern Indians first introduced this medicinal plant to our early fore-fathers and also how to beneficially use it.

For gastric and duodenal ulcers, it should be combined with golden seal, which gives it the proper stimulative effect.

When using as a gargle, it will at first render a stinging sensation, but in a short time it will have an anesthetic effect.

It is important to take internally while treating external maladies.

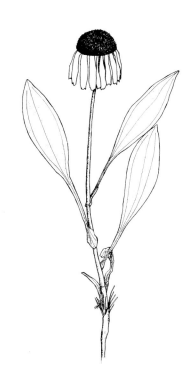

PREPARATION:

DECOCTION (See Section 7 for General Decoction Preparation Information)
STANDARD DECOCTION (Boil for 3 minutes)
Dosage: 1 wineglassful T.I.D. or Q.I.D.

FLUID EXTRACT (See Section 6 for General Fluid Extract Preparation Information)
STANDARD FLUID EXTRACTION (Mix equal parts of the extract with a saturated sugar)
Dosage: 1 dram, 3 to 6 times daily

MEDICINAL PROPERTIES
Alterative
Antiseptic
Tonic
Antibiotic

COMBINATIONS:

For Gastric and Duodenal Ulcers { Purple Cone Flower Golden Seal } In a Standard Decoction

PLANT IDENTIFICATION #43

GUMWEED

Gumplant, Tarweed, Resinweed, Grindelia

GRINDELIA SQUARROSA
Grindelia cuneifolia
Grindelia camporum
Grindelia species

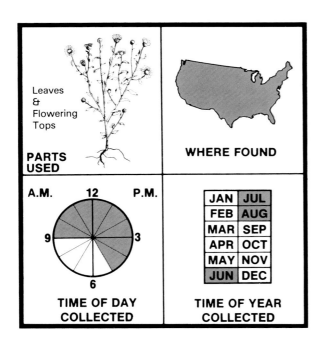

PARTS USED — Leaves & Flowering Tops

WHERE FOUND

TIME OF DAY COLLECTED

TIME OF YEAR COLLECTED

JAN	JUL
FEB	AUG
MAR	SEP
APR	OCT
MAY	NOV
JUN	DEC

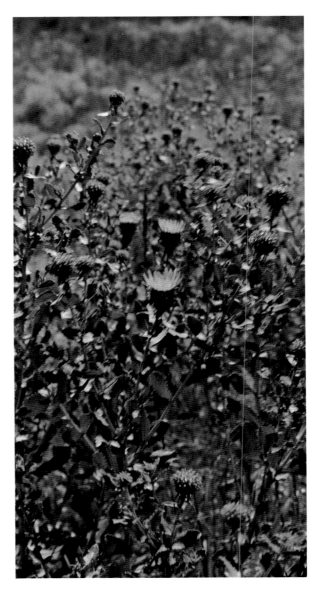

MEDICINAL USES:

- Poison Ivy & Poison Oak Dermatitis
- Impetigo
- Dry Coughs
- Eczema
- Allergenic Dermatitis
- Indolent ulcers

- Coughs & Wheezing
- Asthmatic Chest Tightness (not associated with cardiac problems)

PLANT INFORMATION:

Gumweed is a member of the Sunflower Family (Compositae) and is easily identified by its resinous or gummy leaves and flowering heads.

They are found growing along road-sides and in soils which have been disturbed by construction equipment.

All U.S. species of Gumweed are medicinal.

When applying as a wash for Rhus Poisoning, it should also be taken internally as an infusion. (Or capsulated in powdered form).

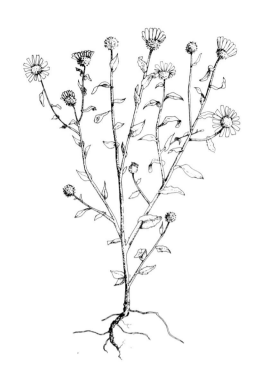

PREPARATION:

INFUSION   (See Section 7 for general infusion preparation information)

MAKE STANDARD INFUSION
As needed for Rhus Poisoning Wash.
Internal use - One wineglassful T.I.D.

POWDER (See Section 8 for general powdering information)

MECHANICAL POWDERING
Capsulate in from 5 to 20 grain quantities.
Dosage: 5 to 40 grains. Q.I.D.

MEDICINAL PROPERTIES

Respiratory Stimulant and
    Expectorant
Dermatological Applicant

PLANT IDENTIFICATION #44

YELLOW CLOVER

Kings Clover, Clover, Yellow Melilot
Sweet Clover, Sweet Lucerne

MELILOTUS OFFICINALIS

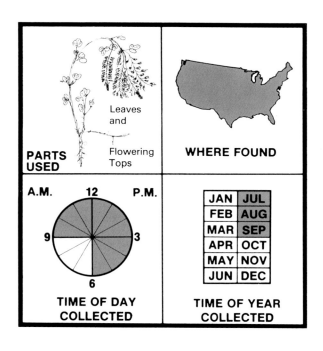

Leaves and Flowering Tops **PARTS USED**	**WHERE FOUND**
TIME OF DAY COLLECTED	JAN/JUL FEB/AUG MAR/SEP APR/OCT MAY/NOV JUN/DEC **TIME OF YEAR COLLECTED**

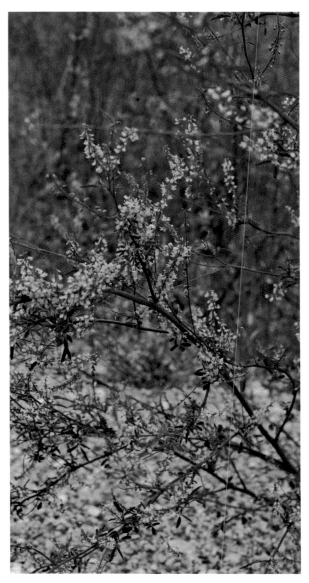

MEDICINAL USES:

- Prolongs prothrombic and coagulation time of the clotting process.

- Idiopathic headaches

- Ovary & uterine pains

- Dysmenorrhea of antispasmodic origin

- Prolongs prothrombic and coagulation time of the clotting process

- Idiopathic headaches

- Ovary & uterine pains

- Dysmenorrhea of antispasmodic origin

PLANT INFORMATION:

Yellow Clover is a member of the Pea Family (Leguminosae). It is found primarily along road cuts and other areas where there has been recent soil disturbance. Oftimes it will even invade home lawns.

Melilotus is used in place of heparin for the treatment of blood clotting - it being an anti-vitamin K agent.

This plant should only be used under a physicians direction. People with a tendency for easy bleeding should not take this plant.

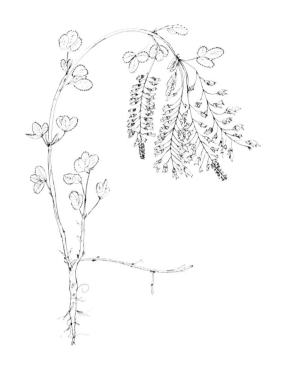

PREPARATION:

INFUSION (See Section 7 for general infusion preparation information)

Boil for 3 minutes, 1 oz. of flowers and leaves in 1 quart of water.
Dosage: 4 ounces T.I.D.

POWDERED PLANT (See Section 8 for general powdering information)

STANDARD POWDERING TECHNIQUE
Dosage: 1 to 50 grains B.I.D.

MEDICINAL PROPERTIES

Nervine
Antispasmodic
Antithrombic

141

PLANT IDENTIFICATION #45

BISTORTA

Snakeweed, Sweet Dock
Dragon wort

POLYGONUM BISTORTOIDES

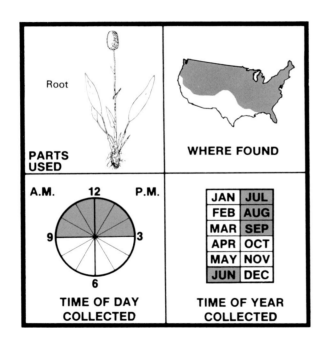

Root **PARTS USED**	**WHERE FOUND**
A.M. 12 P.M. 9 3 6 **TIME OF DAY COLLECTED**	JAN **JUL** FEB **AUG** MAR **SEP** APR OCT MAY NOV **JUN** DEC **TIME OF YEAR COLLECTED**

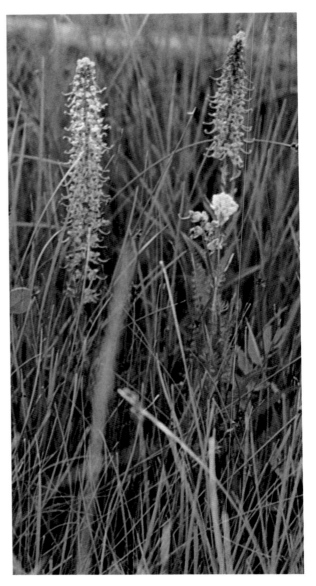

MEDICINAL USES:

- Sores on the gums (Canker sores) Use as a gargle.

- Regulate menstral flow. Use as a douche.

- Leucorrhea

- Stop bleeding cuts & wounds. Apply powdered root directly.

PLANT INFORMATION:

Bistort root is a member of the Buckwheat Family (Polygonaceae). It is found growing at higher elevations (6000 to 9000 feet.) and seems to prefer a moist clay-loam soil. Its "snow-ball" flowering top help one to locate it rather easily.

It is commonly associated with a plant called Elephant Head (Pedicularis) and the sedges (Carex). See photo on opposite page.

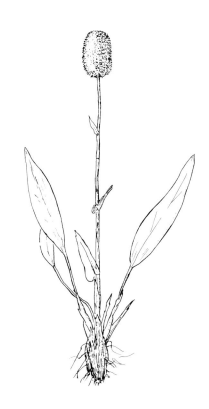

PREPARATION:

DECOCTION (See Section 7 for general decotion preparation information)

STANDARD DECOCTION
Dosage: One wine glass full as needed

POWDERED PLANT (See Section 8 for general powdering information)

STANDARD POWDERING TECHNIQUE
Dosage: 10 to 60 grains or apply directly as needed.

MEDICINAL PROPERTIES
Astringent
Styptic
Alterative

PLANT IDENTIFICATION #46

POTENTELLA
Cinquefoil
Five Fingers
Silverweed

POTENTILLA ANSERINA
Potentilla reptans
Potentilla fruticosa
Potentilla canadensis

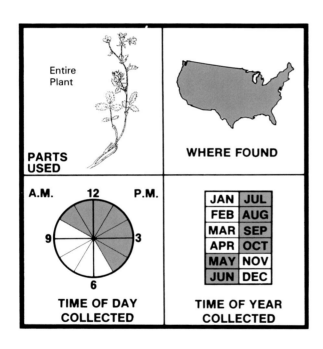

Entire
Plant

PARTS USED

WHERE FOUND

A.M.   12   P.M.

9   3

6

TIME OF DAY COLLECTED

JAN	JUL
FEB	AUG
MAR	SEP
APR	OCT
MAY	NOV
JUN	DEC

TIME OF YEAR COLLECTED

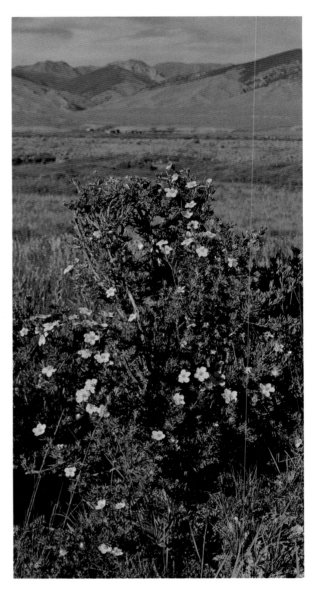

MEDICINAL USES:

- Ague (flu)

- Chills (Recurrent)

- Sore Throat

- Tooth Ache

- Nerve Tonic

- Muscle Spasms

144

PLANT INFORMATION:

Potentilla is a member of the Rose Family (Rosaceae). The flower petals are yellow, and there are many species in this genus. Its distribution is throughout the U.S. and is considered a world-wide plant.

The word Potentilla means ''the little potent one'' indicating its use as a medicinal plant. Besides its value as a nervine and astringent, it is a good diuretic. To ease the discomfort of a sore throat, take the tea with a small amount of honey.

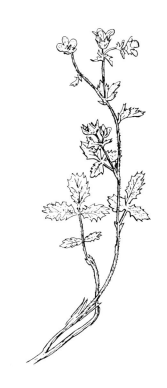

PREPARATION:

INFUSION (See Section 7 for General Infusion Preparation Information)
STANDARD INFUSION
One ounce of chopped leaves and stems in one pint of boiling water, steep for 20 minutes.
Dosage: One wineglassful T.I.D.

TINCTURE (See Section 6 for General Tincture Preparation Information)
(Prepare same as Yarrow)
See Page 113
Dosage: 5 to 10 ggt Q.I.D.

EMERGENCY/DECOCTION
Boil cleaned roots in 2 pints of brown vinegar for about 15 minutes. Cool. Let cooled tea stand in mouth for several minutes.

**MEDICINAL
PROPERTIES**
Tonic
Nervine
Antispasmodic
Astringent

145

PLANT IDENTIFICATION #47

CHICORY

Blue Succory
Hendibeh
Wild Endive
Garden Chicory

CICHORIUM INTYBUS L.

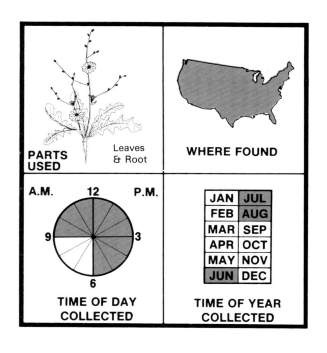

PARTS USED	Leaves & Root	WHERE FOUND
TIME OF DAY COLLECTED		TIME OF YEAR COLLECTED

JAN	JUL
FEB	AUG
MAR	SEP
APR	OCT
MAY	NOV
JUN	DEC

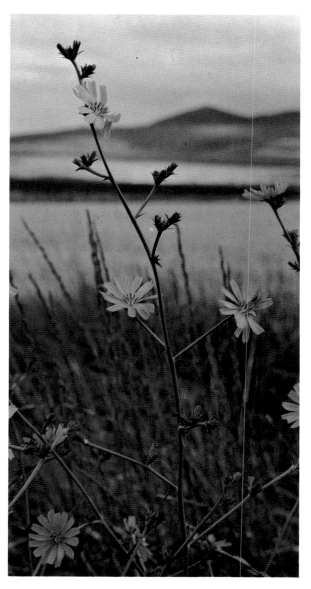

MEDICINAL USES:

- Gout

- Upset Stomach

- Jaundice

PLANT INFORMATION:

Chicory is in the Sunflower Family (Compositae). The best time to collect the leaves is just before anthesis (flowering time). The roots can be collected anytime.

The blanched leaves can be used in salad making, and the roots (boiled or baked) make a good stew enhancer.

The roots can be packed in sand and stored in a "root cellar" with only the top part of the root exposed at the surface. The roots will send forth shoots which make a good salad ingredient.

Chicory roots can be collected, sliced, dried, ground, and used with ground coffee, or in place of coffee when drinking it for medicinal reasons.

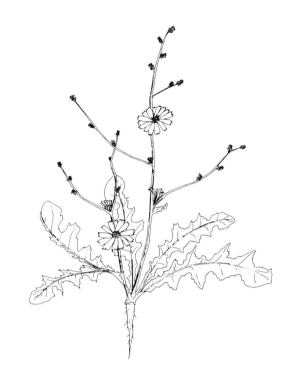

PREPARATION:

DECOCTION (See Section 7 for General Decoction Preparation Information)

1 ounce of root to 1 pint of boiling water.

Dosage: Take wineglassful freely

MEDICINAL PROPERTIES
Diuretic
Laxative
Tonic

PLANT IDENTIFICATION #48

CAYENNE

Guinea Pepper, African Bird Pepper
Chillies, Capsicum, Spanish Pepper

CAPSICUM FASTIGIATUM
Capsicum frutescens

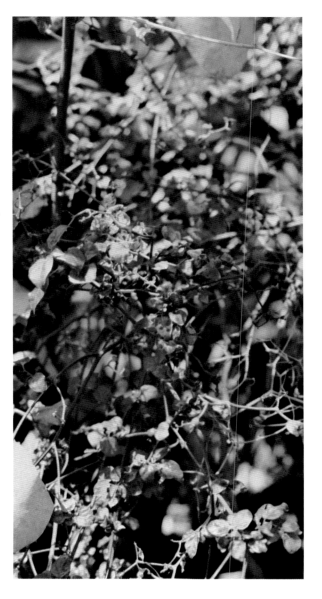

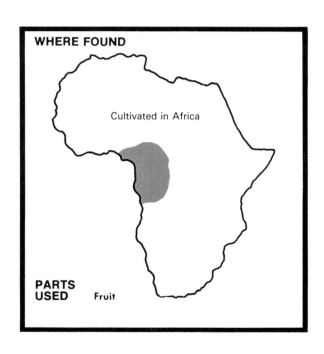

WHERE FOUND

Cultivated in Africa

PARTS USED   Fruit

MEDICINAL USES:

- Removes Excess Mucus Secretions
- Stabilizes or Normalizes Blood Pressure.
- Heart Attacks
- Colds
- Hemorrhage

- Asthmatical Conditions
- Chills
- Flu
- Ulcers
- Coughs
- Circulatory Conditioner
- Tonsillitis

- Profuse Menstrual Hemorrhage

148

PLANT INFORMATION:

Cayenne is a member of the Night Shade Family (Solanaceae). Other plants in this family include; tobacco (Nicotiana), Jimsonweed (Datura), and the Petunia.

It is one of the finest botanicals available and its therapeutic uses should be studied to perfect its application to human needs.*

The best and most effective Cayenne is called African Bird Cayenne. *(Capsicum fastigiatum* and *Capsicum frutescens).*

For people having trouble keeping their feet warm at night, place a small amount of cayenne in the socks and sleep with them on. It will solve the cold feet problem.

Cayenne should be used on a daily basis for its nutritive qualities. It is rich in Vitamin C, A, B_1 and G. Its mineral content includes Calcium, Phosphorus and Iron.

It should be used in conjunction with many other botanicals as a stimulant for there is none its equal.

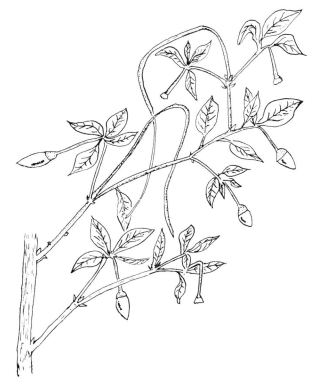

PREPARATION:

INFUSION (See Section 7 for General Infusion preparation information)

STANDARD INFUSION
Dosage: Drink Freely

TINCTURE (See Section 6 for General Tincture Preparation information)

Macerate 2 ounces of Cayenne for 14 days in one quart of 40% alcohol. (Keep warm while soaking).

Dosage: 10 to 14 minims T.I.D.

POWDER (Special Emergency Preparation for profuse menstrual bleeding)

Mix 1 teaspoonful of powdered cayenne in a glass of water or unsweetened juice.

Dosage: Once every twenty minutes.

MEDICINAL PROPERTIES

Stimulant, Carminative
Tonic, Stomachic
Rubefacient, Pungent
Emetic, Astringent
Alterative, Antiseptic
Nutrient, Antispasmodic

*A monograph on the comprehensive therapeutic functions of Cayenne and other Botanicals may be obtained from ROYAL BOTANICAL COMPANY.

PLANT TAXONOMY

Methods and principles of Plant Classification.

Botanists identify plants by comparing or choosing one plant character over another. Flowers, Roots, Leaves, Stems, Shapes, Colors and many more characteristics are compared.

This section will superficially give the reader an idea how to "run down" or to determine one group of plants from another. This same principle applies in determining species of plants.

Our approach will be to compare two seeds and make the comparison choice available to us, and to follow the colored route to the next set of choices.

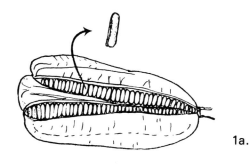

1a.   Seed with a covering. (Example: Peas, cherries, acorns, peaches, apples, etc.)

OR

1b.   Seed without a covering (Example: Ephedra, Pine nuts, Horse tails, etc.)

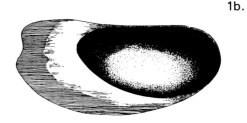

As you become more familiar with plant groups, you will be able to "spot" family characteristics, and then generally by simply using the flowering parts, determine genus and species.

Most Colleges and Universities have excellent Botany Departments. Enrolling in beginning Identification Classes, will greatly increase your knowledge of important plants, and provide important information needed in Plant Classification.

There may be people who know the plants in your area. If they are willing to take you on a little expedition to the fields and mountains, you can learn many times faster than if you stumble through some difficult Botany "Key".

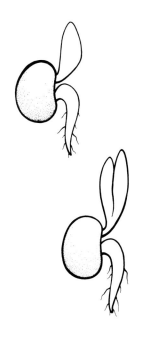

See Page 154

2a. **Sprouted Seed with One-Seed leaf.**
     The Monocotyledons (Mono = one + Cotyledon = seed leaf)

OR   The flowering plants

See Page 156

2b. **Sprouted Seed with Two-Seed leaves.**
     The Dicotyledons (Di = two + Cotyledon = seed leaf)

See Page 152

Angiosperms
(angio = vessel + sperm = seed)

Gymnosperms
(gymno = naked + sperm = seed)

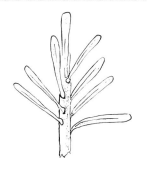

3a. Sprouted seed generally with 3 or more seed leaves.
     Needles single on the branch.

See Page 152

OR   The ''flowerless'' plants

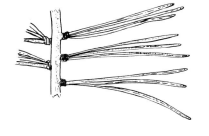

3b. Needles in vascular bundles of 2 or more.

PLANT TAXONOMY

NEEDLE SHAPES

THE GYMNOSPERMS

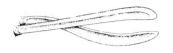

4a.   ABIES (The Firs)

        Needles Flat and Flexible
        Needles point skyward
        Cones not pendulous (sit erect on branch)

     OR

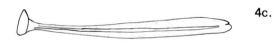

4b.   PICEA (The Spruces)

        Needles Sharp and Single
        Needles Square (in cross-section)
        Spicule (needle nob remains after needle fall)

     OR

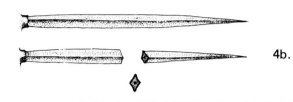

4c.   PSEUDOTSUGA (The Douglas Firs)

        Needles Pedicellate
        Needles flat and delicate
        Cones with 3-lobed bracts

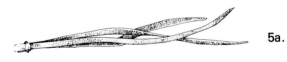

5a.   PINUS (The Pines)

        Needles 2 or more surrounded by
          papery sheath (Fascicle)
        Many of the seed (Nuts) edible.

     OR

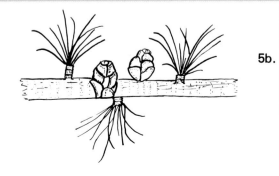

5b.   LARIX (The Larches)

        Needles many and in whorls
        Needles deciduous (drop in the fall of the year)

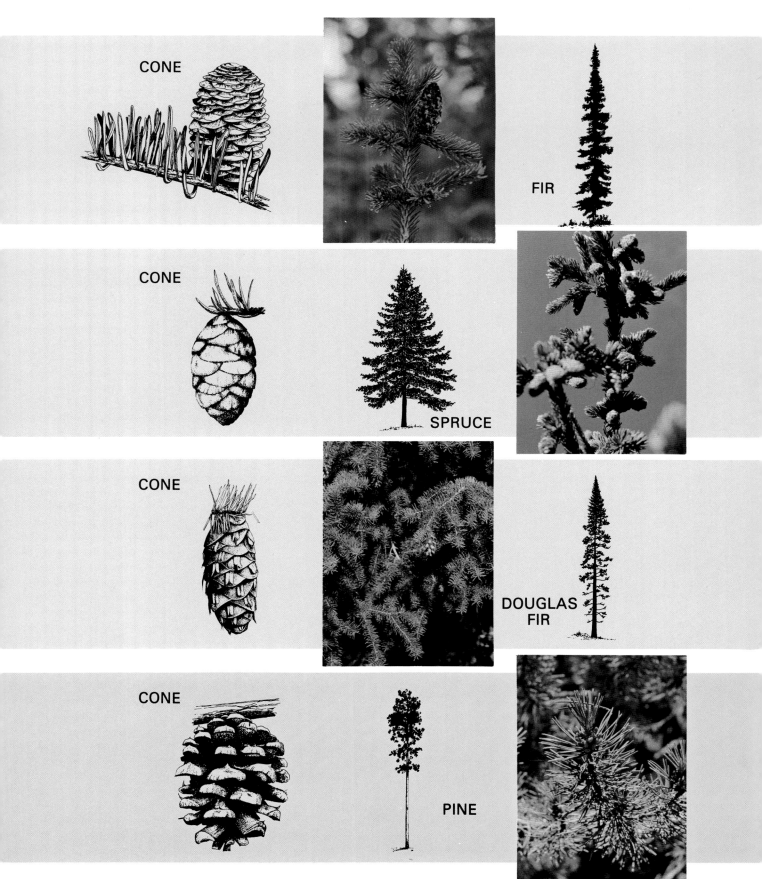

CONE

CONE

FIR

CONE

SPRUCE

CONE

DOUGLAS
FIR

PINE

PLANT TAXONOMY

THE MONOCOTYLEDONS

Characteristics of the Monocots

1. Flower parts (Petals, Sepals, etc. usually in series of three.

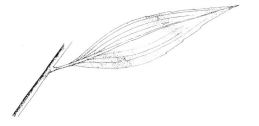

2. Leaf Veins parallel to each other.

6a.   Plants Not Grass-like.

OR

6b.   Plants Grass-like

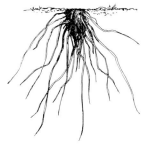

3. Root system fibrous (without a single tap root.

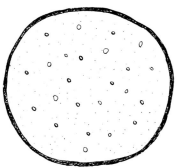

4. Stem with pithy tissue vascular bundles scattered irregularily through the stem tissue.

154

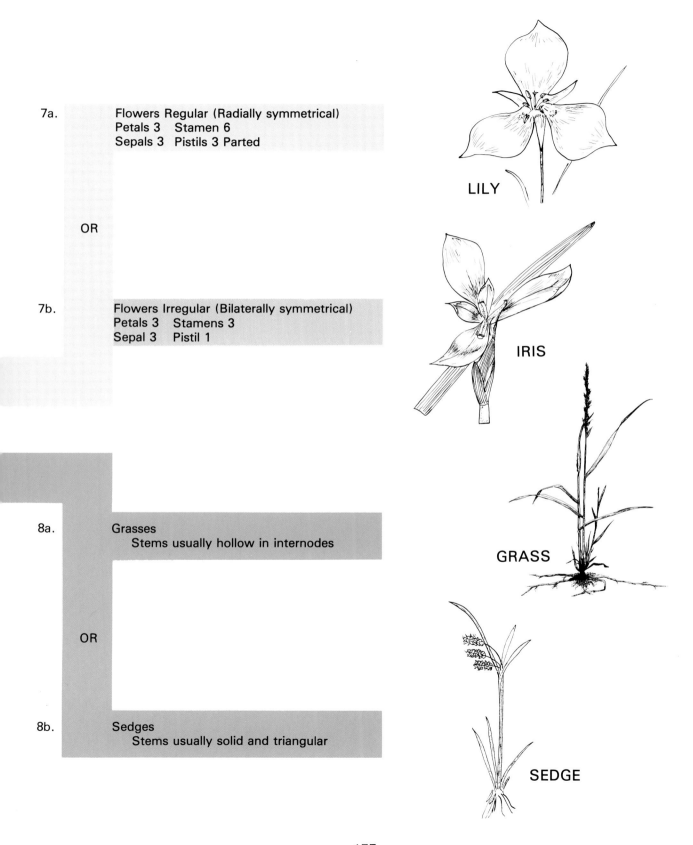

7a.   Flowers Regular (Radially symmetrical)
Petals 3   Stamen 6
Sepals 3   Pistils 3 Parted

LILY

OR

7b.   Flowers Irregular (Bilaterally symmetrical)
Petals 3   Stamens 3
Sepal 3   Pistil 1

IRIS

8a.   Grasses
Stems usually hollow in internodes

GRASS

OR

8b.   Sedges
Stems usually solid and triangular

SEDGE

155

PLANT TAXONOMY

THE DICOTYLEDONS

Characteristics of the Dicots

1. Flower parts arranged in 2's, 4's, or usually 5's.

9a.

2. Leaf veins netted not parallel.

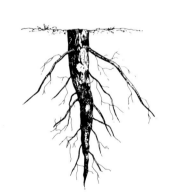

OR

3. Root system characterized by a tap root

9b.

4. Stems with "rings" or vascular bundles in a single cylinder. (as seen in x-section)

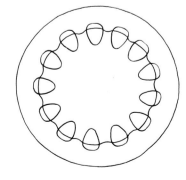

10a. Petals-4. Stamens-4 and 2.
Sepals-4. Fruit-a silique.

COMMON MUSTARD

OR Petals separate
Leaves alternate

10b. Petals-5. Stamens-many with united filaments.
Sepals-5, more or less united. Fruit-a capsule.

HOLLEY HOCK

11a. Petals-5, 2 lipped. Stamens-4, in 2 unequal pairs.
Stems-square. Fruit-4 nutlets.

MINT

OR Petals united
Leaves opposite

11b. Petals-5, usually 2 lipped (not aromatic).
Stamens-4 or 5, one sometimes sterile.
Fruit-a capsule.

PENSTAMON

157

Section X

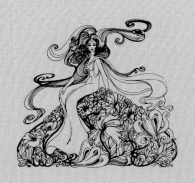

PREPARATION FOR DRAWING SALVE*

INGREDIENTS:

Beeswax - Size of Walnut
Pine (Conifer) Resin - 1 Part (Qt.)
Mutton Tallow - 1 Part (Qt.)

GENERAL USES:

For Blood Poisoning
For Infection (Sores) Both Man and Animal
For Hemorrhoids (External Use)

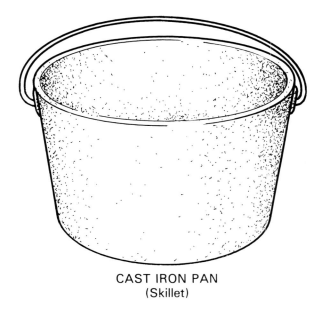

CAST IRON PAN
(Skillet)

PROCEDURE:

(1) Obtain fresh mutton tallow (not beef tallow)

(2) Render out the tallow (melt into an oil condition)

(3) Strain through a loose weaved cloth (an old clean dish towel will do)

(4) Strain into a clean one gallon container for use or for future use. Will store indefinitely without going rancid.

(5) When ready to use: Re-Melt in a cast iron pan (skillet) after mutton is melted turn temperature to low heat or simmer.

(6) Add equal part of pine resin.

CAUTION: DO NOT BOIL
(Keep temperature on low or
simmer once mutton has melted.)

---

(7) Stir until oil and resin are completely blended.

(8) Shave in beeswax (about ¾ of block).

(9) Mix in well by stirring.

(10) Strain again (to remove resin impurities) and pour into a clean gallon container which will serve as a pouring container.

(11) Pour into smaller jars. Pour before salve becomes cool.

(12) Leave to cool and solidify over night - When solidified it is ready to use.

OBTAINING BASIC INGREDIENTS:

MUTTON TALLOW: May be obtained from those who raise sheep or a slaughter house.

PINE GUM OR RESIN: May be obtained from any Pine, Spruce, or Fir Tree as follows:

In late May or early June, Pine Sap Flows.

With a sharp instrument, notch a V-shaped cut into the tree and place a can or other collecting receptacle to catch the bleeding or running resin. Select an older tree for cutting. Pinus monophylla produces excellent gum resins which can be picked from the tree or from the ground.

TREE TRUNK

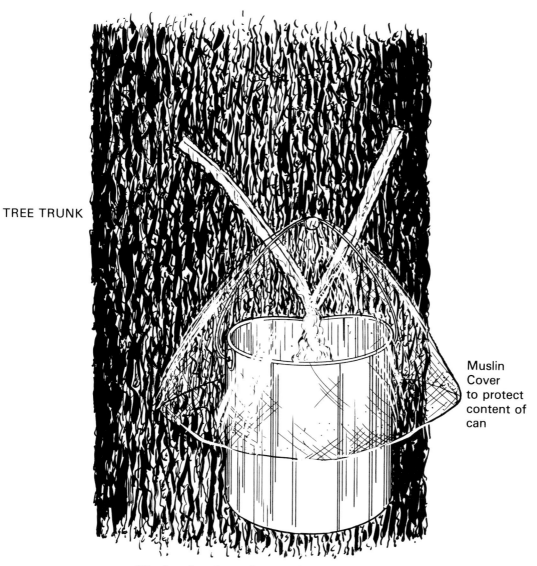

Muslin
Cover
to protect
content of
can

*The formula and procedure was given to the Author by Nona Cassidy of Afton, (Osmond) Wyoming.

161

GENERAL PLANT STUDIES

To become more proficient in the study of medicinal plants, it is desirable to "round-out" your knowledge of some of the more common plants in America and something of their Natural History. This section of the book will list some 66 plants and leave room for you to fill in the data as you find and identify the plant designated by the plant identification number. Below is an example using the plant called wild lettuce or compass plant to show what possibilities can be had with this "field" study section.

Plant data is best acquired by lectures, published sources, college and university botany classes. When possible, travel with a person who can assist you in your desire to learn medicinal plants.

Four catagories of plants are considered:

MEDICINAL - Other plants which are and can be used in the healing arts.

POISONOUS - Plants which can cause poisoning or mechanical harm.

EDIBLE - Plants which can be used for survival.

GENERAL - Plants which are interesting to study.

Floral Formula	**PLANT IDENTIFICATION #115**	FIELD DATA
Petals _____	Scientific Name: *Lactuca scariola*	Date Identified _____
Sepals _____	Common Name: Wild Lettuce (Edible)	Locality _____
Stamens _____		Plant Information:
Pistil _____		
Family _____		

A field note book should be taken along listing some of the following data:
Date of collection
Associated species (other types of plants found growing around or near collected plant)
Where found (where possible list Township, Range, and Section) List county, river
    drainage, exposure to the sun (N.E.S.W.)
Soil type (sandy, loam, clay, etc.)
Flower color at time of collection.

Floral Formula

Petals _____
Sepals _____
Stamens _____
Pistil _____

Family _____

PLANT IDENTIFICATION #49
Amaranthus retroflexus
Red Root (Edible)

FIELD DATA

Date Identified _____
Locality _____
Plant Information:

Floral Formula

Petals _____
Sepals _____
Stamens _____
Pistil _____

Family _____

PLANT IDENTIFICATION #50
Rhus toxidendron
Poison Ivy (Poisonous)

FIELD DATA

Date Identified _____
Locality _____
Plant Information:

Floral Formula

Petals _____
Sepals _____
Stamens _____
Pistil _____

Family _____

PLANT IDENTIFICATION #51
Cynoglossum officinalis
Houndstongue (Medicinal)

FIELD DATA

Date Identified _____
Locality _____
Plant Information:

Floral Formula

Petals _____
Sepals _____
Stamens _____
Pistil _____

Family _____

PLANT IDENTIFICATION #52
Opuntia species
Prickly Pear (Edible)

FIELD DATA

Date Identified _____
Locality _____
Plant Information:

Floral Formula

Petals _____
Sepals _____
Stamens _____
Pistil _____

Family _____

PLANT IDENTIFICATION #53
Lonicera species
Honeysuckle (Medicinal)

FIELD DATA

Date Identified _____
Locality _____
Plant Information:

Floral Formula

Petals _____
Sepals _____
Stamens _____
Pistil _____

Family _____

PLANT IDENTIFICATION #54
Pachystima myrsinities
Mountain Lover (General)

FIELD DATA

Date Identified _____
Locality _____
Plant Information:

PLANT IDENTIFICATION #55

Floral Formula

Petals _____
Sepals _____
Stamens _____
Pistil _____

Salsola kali
Russian Thistle (Edible)

FIELD DATA

Date Identified _____
Locality _____
Plant Information:

Family _____

PLANT IDENTIFICATION #56

Floral Formula

Petals _____
Sepals _____
Stamens _____
Pistil _____

Sarcobatus vermiculatus
Greasewood (Poison-Medicinal)

FIELD DATA

Date Identified _____
Locality _____
Plant Information:

Family _____

PLANT IDENTIFICATION #57

Floral Formula

Petals _____
Sepals _____
Stamens _____
Pistil _____

Rhamnus purshiana
Cascara (Medicinal)

FIELD DATA

Date Identified _____
Locality _____
Plant Information:

Family _____

PLANT IDENTIFICATION #58

Floral Formula

Petals _____
Sepals _____
Stamens _____
Pistil _____

Kochia scoparia
Kochia (General)

FIELD DATA

Date Identified _____
Locality _____
Plant Information:

Family _____

PLANT IDENTIFICATION #59

Floral Formula

Petals _____
Sepals _____
Stamens _____
Pistil _____

Crepis species
Hawk's Beard (Medicinal)

FIELD DATA

Date Identified _____
Locality _____
Plant Information:

Family _____

PLANT IDENTIFICATION #60

Floral Formula

Petals _____
Sepals _____
Stamens _____
Pistil _____

Antennaria species
Pussy Toes (General)

FIELD DATA

Date Identified _____
Locality _____
Plant Information:

Family _____

Floral Formula

Petals _____
Sepals _____
Stamens _____
Pistil _____

PLANT IDENTIFICATION #61
Anaphalis margaritacea
Pearly Everlasting (Medicinal)

FIELD DATA

Date Identified _____
Locality _____
Plant Information:

Family _____

Floral Formula

Petals _____
Sepals _____
Stamens _____
Pistil _____

PLANT IDENTIFICATION #62
Chimaphilia unbellata
Pippissewa (Medicinal)

FIELD DATA

Date Identified _____
Locality _____
Plant Information:

Family _____

Floral Formula

Petals _____
Sepals _____
Stamens _____
Pistil _____

PLANT IDENTIFICATION #63
Balsamorrhiza species
Balsamroot (Edible)

FIELD DATA

Date Identified _____
Locality _____
Plant Information:

Family _____

Floral Formula

Petals _____
Sepals _____
Stamens _____
Pistil _____

PLANT IDENTIFICATION #64
Centauria cyanus
Knapweed (General)

FIELD DATA

Date Identified _____
Locality _____
Plant Information:

Family _____

Floral Formula

Petals _____
Sepals _____
Stamens _____
Pistil _____

PLANT IDENTIFICATION #65
Chrysothamnus species
Rabbit Brush (General)

FIELD DATA

Date Identified _____
Locality _____
Plant Information:

Family _____

Floral Formula

Petals _____
Sepals _____
Stamens _____
Pistil _____

PLANT IDENTIFICATION #66
Erigeron canadensis
Fleabane (Medicinal)

FIELD DATA

Date Identified _____
Locality _____
Plant Information:

Family _____

Floral Formula	**PLANT IDENTIFICATION #67**	FIELD DATA
Petals _____ Sepals _____ Stamens _____ Pistil _____ Family _____	*Conium maculata* Poison Hemlock (Poison)	Date Identified _____ Locality _____ Plant Information:

Floral Formula	**PLANT IDENTIFICATION #68**	FIELD DATA
Petals _____ Sepals _____ Stamens _____ Pistil _____ Family _____	*Salidago species* Golden Rod (Medicinal)	Date Identified _____ Locality _____ Plant Information:

Floral Formula	**PLANT IDENTIFICATION #69**	FIELD DATA
Petals _____ Sepals _____ Stamens _____ Pistil _____ Family _____	*Tragopogon species* Goat'sbeard (Edible)	Date Identified _____ Locality _____ Plant Information:

Floral Formula	**PLANT IDENTIFICATION #70**	FIELD DATA
Petals _____ Sepals _____ Stamens _____ Pistil _____ Family _____	*Brassica nigra* Mustard (Medicinal)	Date Identified _____ Locality _____ Plant Information:

Floral Formula	**PLANT IDENTIFICATION #71**	FIELD DATA
Petals _____ Sepals _____ Stamens _____ Pistil _____ Family _____	*Tetradymia species* Horsebrush (Poisonous)	Date Identified _____ Locality _____ Plant Information:

Floral Formula	**PLANT IDENTIFICATION #72**	FIELD DATA
Petals _____ Sepals _____ Stamens _____ Pistil _____ Family _____	*Convallaria majalis* Lily-of-the Valley (Medicinal)	Date Identified _____ Locality _____ Plant Information:

Floral Formula

Petals _____
Sepals _____
Stamens _____
Pistil _____

Family _____

PLANT IDENTIFICATION #73
Dipsacus sylvestris
Teasel (General)

FIELD DATA
Date Identified _____
Locality _____
Plant Information:

Floral Formula

Petals _____
Sepals _____
Stamens _____
Pistil _____

Family _____

PLANT IDENTIFICATION #74
Artemesia absinthium
Wormwood (Medicinal)

FIELD DATA
Date Identified _____
Locality _____
Plant Information:

Floral Formula

Petals _____
Sepals _____
Stamens _____
Pistil _____

Family _____

PLANT IDENTIFICATION #75
Marrumbium vulgare
Horehound (Medicinal)

FIELD DATA
Date Identified _____
Locality _____
Plant Information:

Floral Formula

Petals _____
Sepals _____
Stamens _____
Pistil _____

Family _____

PLANT IDENTIFICATION #76
Salvia officinalis
Garden Sage (Medicinal)

FIELD DATA
Date Identified _____
Locality _____
Plant Information:

Floral Formula

Petals _____
Sepals _____
Stamens _____
Pistil _____

Family _____

PLANT IDENTIFICATION #77
Lithosperma species
Stoneseed (Medicinal)

FIELD DATA
Date Identified _____
Locality _____
Plant Information:

Floral Formula

Petals _____
Sepals _____
Stamens _____
Pistil _____

Family _____

PLANT IDENTIFICATION #78
Glycyrrhiza species
Wild Licorice (Edible)

FIELD DATA
Date Identified _____
Locality _____
Plant Information:

Floral Formula	**PLANT IDENTIFICATION #79**	FIELD DATA
Petals _____ Sepals _____ Stamens _____ Pistil _____	*Poliomintha incana* Purple Sage (General)	Date Identified _____ Locality _____ Plant Information:
Family _____		

Floral Formula	**PLANT IDENTIFICATION #80**	FIELD DATA
Petals _____ Sepals _____ Stamens _____ Pistil _____	*Quercus species* Nutgalls (Medicinal)	Date Identified _____ Locality _____ Plant Information:
Family _____		

Floral Formula	**PLANT IDENTIFICATION #81**	FIELD DATA
Petals _____ Sepals _____ Stamens _____ Pistil _____	*Lupinus species* Lupine (General)	Date Identified _____ Locality _____ Plant Information:
Family _____		

Floral Formula	**PLANT IDENTIFICATION #82**	FIELD DATA
Petals _____ Sepals _____ Stamens _____ Pistil _____	*Hyoscyamus niger* Henbane (Poison-Medicinal)	Date Identified _____ Locality _____ Plant Information:
Family _____		

Floral Formula	**PLANT IDENTIFICATION #83**	FIELD DATA
Petals _____ Sepals _____ Stamens _____ Pistil _____	*Impatiens pallida* Touch-me-not (Medicinal)	Date Identified _____ Locality _____ Plant Information:
Family _____		

Floral Formula	**PLANT IDENTIFICATION #84**	FIELD DATA
Petals _____ Sepals _____ Stamens _____ Pistil _____	*Forsythia species* Forsythia (General)	Date Identified _____ Locality _____ Plant Information:
Family _____		

Floral Formula

Petals _____
Sepals _____
Stamens _____
Pistil _____

PLANT IDENTIFICATION #85
Oenothera species
Evening Primrose (General)

FIELD DATA

Date Identified _____
Locality _____
Plant Information:

Family _____

Floral Formula

Petals _____
Sepals _____
Stamens _____
Pistil _____

PLANT IDENTIFICATION #86
Plox species
Phlox (General)

FIELD DATA

Date Identified _____
Locality _____
Plant Information:

Family _____

Floral Formula

Petals _____
Sepals _____
Stamens _____
Pistil _____

PLANT IDENTIFICATION #87
Eriogonum species
Umbrella Plant (Medicinal)

FIELD DATA

Date Identified _____
Locality _____
Plant Information:

Family _____

Floral Formula

Petals _____
Sepals _____
Stamens _____
Pistil _____

PLANT IDENTIFICATION #88
Urtica species
Stinging Nettle (Medicinal)

FIELD DATA

Date Identified _____
Locality _____
Plant Information:

Family _____

Floral Formula

Petals _____
Sepals _____
Stamens _____
Pistil _____

PLANT IDENTIFICATION #89
Wyethia species
Mule's Ears (Medicinal)

FIELD DATA

Date Identified _____
Locality _____
Plant Information:

Family _____

Floral Formula

Petals _____
Sepals _____
Stamens _____
Pistil _____

PLANT IDENTIFICATION #90
Delphinium species
Columbine (General)

FIELD DATA

Date Identified _____
Locality _____
Plant Information:

Family _____

Floral Formula

PLANT IDENTIFICATION #91

Amelanchier species
Service berry (Edible)

FIELD DATA

Petals _____
Sepals _____
Stamens _____
Pistil _____

Date Identified _____
Locality _____
Plant Information:

Family _____

Floral Formula

PLANT IDENTIFICATION #92

Cercocarpus species
Mountain Mahogany (General)

FIELD DATA

Petals _____
Sepals _____
Stamens _____
Pistil _____

Date Identified _____
Locality _____
Plant Information:

Family _____

Floral Formula

PLANT IDENTIFICATION #93

Fragaria americana
Wild Strawberry (Edible)

FIELD DATA

Petals _____
Sepals _____
Stamens _____
Pistil _____

Date Identified _____
Locality _____
Plant Information:

Family _____

Floral Formula

PLANT IDENTIFICATION #94

Heuchera species
Alum root (Medicinal)

FIELD DATA

Petals _____
Sepals _____
Stamens _____
Pistil _____

Date Identified _____
Locality _____
Plant Information:

Family _____

Floral Formula

PLANT IDENTIFICATION #95

Ribes species
Wild Current (Edible)

FIELD DATA

Petals _____
Sepals _____
Stamens _____
Pistil _____

Date Identified _____
Locality _____
Plant Information:

Family _____

Floral Formula

PLANT IDENTIFICATION #96

Castilleja species
Indian Paintbrush (General)

FIELD DATA

Petals _____
Sepals _____
Stamens _____
Pistil _____

Date Identified _____
Locality _____
Plant Information:

Family _____

Floral Formula

PLANT IDENTIFICATION #97

Pedicularis species

Elephant Head (Medicinal)

Petals _____
Sepals _____
Stamens _____
Pistil _____

Family _____

FIELD DATA

Date Identified _____
Locality _____
Plant Information:

Floral Formula

PLANT IDENTIFICATION #98

Penstemon species

Beardtongue (General)

Petals _____
Sepals _____
Stamens _____
Pistil _____

Family _____

FIELD DATA

Date Identified _____
Locality _____
Plant Information:

Floral Formula

PLANT IDENTIFICATION #99

Digitalis purpurea

Foxglove (Medicinal)

Petals _____
Sepals _____
Stamens _____
Pistil _____

Family _____

FIELD DATA

Date Identified _____
Locality _____
Plant Information:

Floral Formula

PLANT IDENTIFICATION #100

Datura species

Jimsonweed (Poison-Medicinal)

Petals _____
Sepals _____
Stamens _____
Pistil _____

Family _____

FIELD DATA

Date Identified _____
Locality _____
Plant Information:

Floral Formula

PLANT IDENTIFICATION #101

Scripus species

Bulrush (Edible)

Petals _____
Sepals _____
Stamens _____
Pistil _____

Family _____

FIELD DATA

Date Identified _____
Locality _____
Plant Information:

Floral Formula

PLANT IDENTIFICATION #102

Typha species

Cattail (Edible)

Petals _____
Sepals _____
Stamens _____
Pistil _____

Family _____

FIELD DATA

Date Identified _____
Locality _____
Plant Information:

PLANT IDENTIFICATION #103

Floral Formula

Petals _____
Sepals _____
Stamens _____
Pistil _____

Family _____

Elymus species
Giant Wild Rye (Edible)

FIELD DATA

Date Identified _____
Locality _____
Plant Information:

PLANT IDENTIFICATION #104

Floral Formula

Petals _____
Sepals _____
Stamens _____
Pistil _____

Family _____

Phragmites communis
Common Reed (General)

FIELD DATA

Date Identified _____
Locality _____
Plant Information:

PLANT IDENTIFICATION #105

Floral Formula

Petals _____
Sepals _____
Stamens _____
Pistil _____

Family _____

Stipa species
Needle-and-thread grass (Poisonous)

FIELD DATA

Date Identified _____
Locality _____
Plant Information:

PLANT IDENTIFICATION #106

Floral Formula

Petals _____
Sepals _____
Stamens _____
Pistil _____

Family _____

Zygadenus paniculatus
Death Camas (Poisonous)

FIELD DATA

Date Identified _____
Locality _____
Plant Information:

PLANT IDENTIFICATION #107

Floral Formula

Petals _____
Sepals _____
Stamens _____
Pistil _____

Family _____

Bromus brizaeformis
Rattlesnake Brome (General)

FIELD DATA

Date Identified _____
Locality _____
Plant Information:

PLANT IDENTIFICATION #108

Floral Formula

Petals _____
Sepals _____
Stamens _____
Pistil _____

Family _____

Hackelia species
Stickseed (General)

FIELD DATA

Date Identified _____
Locality _____
Plant Information:

172

FIELD NOTES/LABORATORY NOTES

NUTRITION WITH THE BOTANICAL NITRILOSIDES (Vitamin B -17)

No botanical work of this nature would be complete without supplying information regarding which plants contain Vitamin B-17, or "Laetrile". Cancer is one of the most dreaded and deadly diseases of our time and is steadily on the increase. Important studies prove that most cancers result from nutritional deficiencies and that by eating food rich in Vitamin B-17 the cancer trends can be reversed and even eliminated. A fresh and mostly uncooked vegetable diet, with a decrease of meat consumption, is indicated for our western civilization as a step in the right direction.

FOODS CONTAINING NITRILOSIDES (Partial List)

A.
Cranberries (Scandinavian types preferred)
Apples including their seeds (chewed)
Peach and Prune kernels
Apricot kernels (One of the best sources - 1 kernel for each 10 pounds of body weight)
Strawberries
Raspberries
Boysenberries
Huckleberries
Blackberries
Plums
Cherry kernels
Elderberries

B.
Millet (can be ground and mixed with whole wheat flour to make bread)
Buckwheat
Alfalfa sprouts
Wheat grass (juices)
Bamboo shoots (Chinese Foods)
Spinach
Water cress
Lentils
Flax seeds
Lima beans
Mung beans (and sprouts)
Garbanzo beans
Cassava
Yams
Fava beans

C.
Cashews (raw)
Pecans (raw)
Macademia nuts
Filbert nuts (raw)

For therapeutic amounts of Vitamin B-17, information concerning sources and supply can be obtained from ROYAL BOTANICAL COMPANY, P.O. Box 2054, Pocatello, Idaho 83201. This company also has information on other botanical preparations.

NUTRITION WITH THE BOTANICAL PANGAMIC ACID (Vitamin B-15)

This vitamin was discovered by one of the great scientists of the century. Its natural sources include rice bran and brewers yeast, and as the name indicates (Pan = all + gamic = seeds), it is found in most plant seeds. It is used in conjunction with Vitamins A, C, E, B-17, and enzymes in the metabolic treatment of cancer.

THERAPEUTIC USES OF PANGAMIC ACID (Partial List)

- Eliminates Hypoxia (insufficient supply of oxygen in cells and tissues).

- Enables cells to effectively respire.

- Slows down the aging process and enhances cyto-functioning.

- It is a natural chelating agent.

- Increases energy levels in the body, and strengthens the bodies' immune system.

- Great aide to recovering heart attack patients.

- Lowers blood pressure.

- Normalizes blood cholesterol levels.

- Useful in the treatment of chronic alcoholism.

- A great liver detoxifier.

- Useful in the treatment of rheumatic heart disease, myocarditis, etc.

- Effective in treating atherosclerosis and emphysema.

- Treatment of chronic hepatitis and primary stages of cirrhosis.

- Treatment for diabetes.

For therapeutic amounts of Vitamin B-15, information concerning sources and supply can be obtained from ROYAL BOTANICAL COMPANY, P.O. Box 2054, Pocatello, Idaho 83201

WEIGHTS AND MEASURES

Metric	Approximate Apothecary Equivalents	Metric	Approximate Apothecary Equivalents	Metric	Approximate Apothecary Equivalents
30 Gm.	1 ounce	0.2 Gm.	3 grains	4 mg.	1/15 grain
15 Gm.	4 drams	0.15 Gm.	2½ grains	3 mg.	1/20 grain
10 Gm.	2½ drams	0.12 Gm.	2 grains	2 mg.	1/30 grain
7.5 Gm.	2 drams	0.1 Gm.	1½ grains	1.5 mg.	1/40 grain
6 Gm.	90 grains	75 mg.	1¼ grains	1.2 mg.	1/50 grain
5 Gm.	75 grains	60 mg.	1 grain	1 mg.	1/60 grain
4 Gm.	60 grains (1 dram)	50 mg.	¾ grain	0.8 mg.	1/80 grain
3 Gm.	45 grains	40 mg.	⅔ grain	0.6 mg.	1/100 grain
2 Gm.	30 grains (½ dram)	30 mg.	½ grain	0.5 mg.	1/120 grain
1.5 Gm.	22 grains	25 mg.	⅜ grain	0.4 mg.	1/150 grain
1 Gm.	15 grains	20 mg.	⅓ grain	0.3 mg.	1/200 grain
0.75 Gm.	12 grains	15 mg.	¼ grain	0.25 mg.	1/250 grain
0.6 Gm.	10 grains	12 mg.	⅕ grain	0.2 mg.	1/300 grain
0.5 Gm.	7½ grains	10 mg.	⅙ grain	0.15 mg.	1/400 grain
0.4 Gm.	6 grains	8 mg.	⅛ grain	0.12 mg.	1/500 grain
0.3 Gm.	5 grains	6 mg.	1/10 grain	0.1 mg.	1/600 grain
0.25 Gm.	4 grains	5 mg.	1/12 grain		

NOTE: A milliliter (ml.) is the approximate equivalent of a cubic centimeter (cc.).

APOTHECARIES

1 dram = 60 grains or ⅛ of an ounce

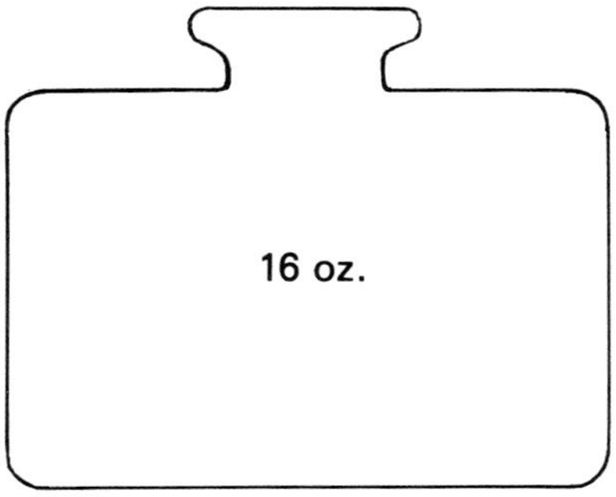

16 ounces = 1 pound

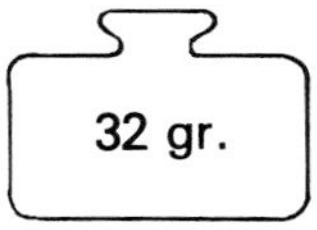

32 grams = 1 ounce

1 milligram = 1/1000 gram

SOLID WEIGHT— LIQUID WEIGHT
1 gram is equal to 1 cc of water at sea level at 4°

* * * * * 15 grains = 1 gram or 1000 milligrams

* 1 grain = 60 milligrams

WEIGHTS AND MEASURES

LIQUIDS

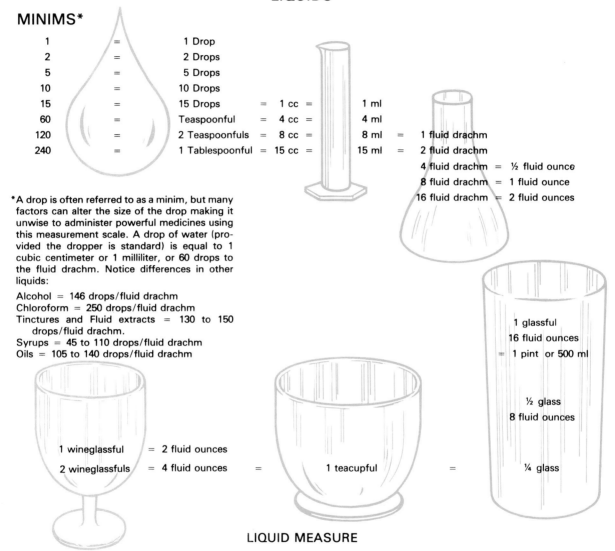

MINIMS*

1	=	1 Drop
2	=	2 Drops
5	=	5 Drops
10	=	10 Drops
15	=	15 Drops	= 1 cc =	1 ml
60	=	Teaspoonful	= 4 cc =	4 ml
120	=	2 Teaspoonfuls	= 8 cc =	8 ml	= 1 fluid drachm
240	=	1 Tablespoonful	= 15 cc =	15 ml	= 2 fluid drachm

4 fluid drachm = ½ fluid ounce
8 fluid drachm = 1 fluid ounce
16 fluid drachm = 2 fluid ounces

*A drop is often referred to as a minim, but many factors can alter the size of the drop making it unwise to administer powerful medicines using this measurement scale. A drop of water (provided the dropper is standard) is equal to 1 cubic centimeter or 1 milliliter, or 60 drops to the fluid drachm. Notice differences in other liquids:

Alcohol = 146 drops/fluid drachm
Chloroform = 250 drops/fluid drachm
Tinctures and Fluid extracts = 130 to 150 drops/fluid drachm.
Syrups = 45 to 110 drops/fluid drachm
Oils = 105 to 140 drops/fluid drachm

1 glassful
16 fluid ounces
= 1 pint or 500 ml

½ glass
8 fluid ounces

1 wineglassful = 2 fluid ounces
2 wineglassfuls = 4 fluid ounces = 1 teacupful = ¼ glass

LIQUID MEASURE

Metric	Approximate Apothecary Equivalents		Metric	Approximate Apothecary Equivalents		Metric	Approximate Apothecary Equivalents	
1000 ml.	1	quart	10 ml.	2½	fluid drams	0.5 ml.	8	minims
750 ml.	1½	pints	8 ml.	2	fluid drams	0.3 ml.	5	minims
500 ml.	1	pint	5 ml.	1¼	fluid drams	0.25 ml.	4	minims
250 ml.	8	fluid ounces	4 ml.	1	fluid dram	0.2 ml.	3	minims
200 ml.	7	fluid ounces	3 ml.	45	minims	0.1 ml.	1½	minims
100 ml.	3½	fluid ounces	2 ml.	30	minims	0.06 ml.	1	minim
50 ml.	1¾	fluid ounces	1 ml.	15	minims	0.05 ml.	¾	minim
30 ml.	1	fluid ounce	0.75 ml.	12	minims	0.03 ml.	½	minim
15 ml.	4	fluid drams	0.6 ml.	10	minims			

GLOSSARY

ADRENAL DYSFUNCTION - Abnormal functioning of the adrenal gland.

AGUE - A chill - Sometimes referring to malarial fever.

ALIMENTARY CANAL CATARRH - Inflammation of the mucous membrane of the head, throat, stomach, and the lower intestines.

ALTERATIVE - Blood purifiers. Remedies which correct impurities of the blood.

AMENORRHEA - Absence of, or abnormal stoppage of the menses or menstrual periods.

ANESTHETIC - A substance or drug that is used to abolish pain.

ANODYNE - A pain reliever.

ANTHELMINTHIC - Something that destroys internal parasites or worms.

ANTIBIOTIC - Generally refers to an agent that is destructive to bacteria.

ANTIHEMORRHAGIC - An agent which stops bleeding.

ANTIHISTIMINE - An agent which counteracts the capillary dilating action histamine and causes the capillaries to constrict thus reducing the amounts of mucous secretions.

ANTIPERIODIC - An agent which controls malarial recurrences.

ANTISCORBUTIC - An effective agent in the treatment and prevention of Scurvy.

ANTISEPTIC - A substance or medicinal agent which prevents or destroys micro-organisms responsible for decay or putrefication.

ANTITHROMBIC - A general tems for a naturally occuring substance which neutralizes the ability of thrombin, limiting blood coagulation.

ANTITUSSIVE - Relieving or preventing coughs.

APERIENT - A mild or gentle purgative.

AROMATIC - A substance with a fragrant smell, and which possesses stimulant factors.

ARTERIOSCLEROSIS - Hardening and thickening of the walls of the arterioles.

ARTHRITIS - Inflammation of the joints.

ARTHROPOD - An animal with jointed appendages (legs) and hard body covering (exoskeleton). Spiders, insects, centipedes, etc.

ASTHMATICS - Wheezing, coughing, and bronchial contractions resulting in dyspnea (difficult or labored breathing).

ASTRINGENTS - Agents which cause the tissue to contract. Astringents are vasoconstrictors, inhibiting the bleeding process.

ATONIC DYSPEPSIA - Lack of strength in the digestive organs.

ATONIC LEUKORRHEA - Loss of vaginal tone accompanied by a white viscid discharge from the vaginal area.

BACTERIOCIDE - An agent which destroys bacteria.

B.I.D. - An abbreviation for the Latin *bis in die* - twice a day.

BRONCHITIS - Inflammation of the bronchial tubes.

CANKER - A moist open sore, mainly of the lips or gums.

CARBUNCLE - A mass of dead cells infecting layers of the surface tissue. Usually caused by the bacterium *Staphylococcus aureus.*

CARDIAC DROPSY - An abnormal accumulation of serous fluid in the heart tissue.

CARMINATIVE - Relieves stomach or intestinal gases.

CATABOLIC WASTES - Waste materials which are produced by the functioning of body chemistry.

CATARRHAL - A word used more frequently by herbalists and Natural Healers to describe the inflammation and free secretions of the mucous membranes.

CHOLERETIC - An agent which stimulates bile excretion by the liver.

COAGULATION - The process of forming a blood clot.

COMMINUTED - To break or crush into small particles.

CONJUNCTIVITIS - Inflammation of the thin transparent tissue which surrounds the eyeball. Pink-eye.

CONVULSIONS - A violent, involuntary contraction of the voluntary muscles.

COROLLA - A term applied to the combined petals of a flower.

COSMOPOLITAN - Not local, having world-wide implications.

COUNTERIRRITANT - A substance or irritation which is intended to relieve some other irritation or pain.

CRADLE CAP - The build-up of soft tissue on or near the anterior soft-spot.

CROUP - An obstruction of the larynx caused by infection and catarrhal discharge.

CYSTITIS - Inflammation of the Urinary Bladder.

D.T.'s - Delirium tremens. A variety of mental disturbances manifested by trembling and mental anxiety usually associated with alcoholism.

DESQUAMATION - The shedding of epithelial skin - usually in scales or sheets.

DEMULCENT - An agent which soothes irritated or inflammed surfaces. A mucilagenous medicine or application.

DERMATITIS - Inflammation or eruptions of the skin.

DERMATOLOGICAL APPLICANT - A substance applied to the skin surfaces for general beneficial purposes.

DESSICATION - To promote drying - loss of moisture due to the drying process.

DETERGENT - An agent which purifies or cleanses.

DETOXIFIER - A substance which removes or neutralizes the properties of a poison.

DEVONIAN - A time period of the Paleozoic Era - between the Silurian and Mississippian periods and geologically recorded in hundreds of millions of years.

DIABETES - A disease condition in which the normal body insulin out-put is in dysfunction.

DIAPHORETIC - An agent which promotes perspiration, or unusually profuse sweating.

DIGESTANT - An agent which assists or stimulates digestion.

DIPTEROUS INSECTS - Flying bugs with two *(di =* two + *ptera =* wings) wings. Mosquitoes, House Flies, etc.

DIURETIC - An agent which promotes the flow of urine.

DRACHMS - An older meaning in the apothecaries' system of measurement equivalent to 60 grains (⅛th of an ounce), more commonly called a dram.

DROPSY - The abnormal accumulation of serous fluid in the cellular tissues or in the body cavity.

DUODENAL ULCERS - Cellular or tissue break-down in the first or proximal portions of the small intestine (Latin *duode 'bi =* 12 at a time, so called because it is about 12 fingerbreadths in length)

DUODENITIS - Inflammation of the small intestines (between the lower end of the stomach (pylorus) and the jejunum.

DYSENTARY - A condition marked by inflammation of the intestine (usually the colon) with feces containing blood and mucous.

DYSPEPSIA - An impairment of the digestive processes.

DYSMENORRHEA - Painful menstruation.

DYSURIA - Painful or difficult urination.

ECZEMA - A inflammatory skin disease with lesions and watery discharges which usually develops scales or incrustations.

ELLIPTIC - Describes the leaf shape, as in the form of an ellipse. (about 1 ½ times as long as broad).

EMETIC - An agent which causes or brings on the act of vomiting.

EMMENOGOGUE - An agent that induces menstruation.

EMOLLIENT - An agent which softens or soothes the skin - or soothes an internal surface.

EMPHYSEMA - A morbid condition of the lungs in which they loose their natural elasticity and forced breathing is necessary to fill oxygen requirements.

ENDOCARDITIS - Inflammation of the inside heart membrane.

EPILEPSY - A disease characterized by recurring loss of consciousness, involuntary muscle movements, and psychic disturbances.

EXCESSIVE MENSES - An over abundant bloody discharge during regular menstruation.

EXPECTORANT - An agent that helps the ejection of mucous from the lungs and bronchial tubes.

EXTERNAL ABSCESSES - A localized collection of pus in a cavity formed by the break down of tissue on or beneath the skin surface.

FEBRIFUGE- An agent or substance which reduces body fever.

FEMALE CLIMACTERIC - The critical or turning point in a woman's life in which the psychic and somatic changes occur at the termination of the normal reproductive period.

FERMENTATIVE DYSPEPSIA - A condition in which the fermentative process interfers with normal digestion.

FLATULENT - Distended (filled) with stomach or intestingal gases.

FLORAL RECEPTACLE - The part of the flower to which the petals, sepals, and other flower parts are attached.

FLUID EXTRACT - A liquid preparation of a vegetable drug containing alcohol as a solvent and preservative. Preparation ratio - 1 gram of plant material to 1 ml. of solvent.

FOMENTATION - This word is oftimes used to mean a poultice. It specifically refers to the substance applied.

GASTRITIS - Inflammation of the stomach.

GESTATION - The period of development from the time the ovum (egg) is fertilized to the time of birth.

GLEET - A form of gonorrhea.

GENITALS - The male and female organs of reproduction.

GRANULATED - A grain-sized mass or formation. For example- as a grated carrot or potato.

GRAVEL - The coarse concretions (solid mass) of mineral salts formed in the kidney and/or bladder.

GTT - g.t.t. - Abbreviation for drop. Minim.

HEMORRHAGE - A large escape of blood from the vessels; bleeding.

HEMORRHOIDS - Varicose blood vessels of the interior anal or rectal cavity. Piles.

HEMOSTATIC - An agent which checks or stops the flow of blood.

HEPATIC - Pertains to the liver and its proper functions.

HERPES - An inflammatory skin disease with small vesicles formed in clusters. (Cold sore is an example).

HYDROPHOBIA - Old word for the disease, Rabies.

HYGROSCOPIC - The tendency or ability of a substance to absorb moisture from the air.

IDIOPATHIC HEADACHE - Headache of unknown origin or cause.

IMPETIGO - A bacterial inflammatory skin disease.

INDOLENT ULCERS - Ulcers which cause only a little pain or discomfort.

INFUSION - Another term for a tea. Extraction of a medicinal property by using hot or sometimes cold water.

INSOMNIA - The inability to sleep; abnormal wakefulness.

INTERCOSTAL NEURALGIA - Pain in the ribs or in the side.

INTERMITTENT FEVER - A fever that is elevated for a period of time, and then temporarily returns to normal; reoccuring high and normal temperatures.

JAUNDICE - A condition of many origins in which there is a deposit of bile pigments in the skin and mucous membranes resulting in a yellow appearance.

LACTATION - The process of giving milk. Suckling.

LANCEOLATE - Refers to the leaf shape being lance-shaped. Four to six times as long as it is broad. Broadest at the base.

LAXATIVE - An agent that acts to promote the evacuation of the bowels.

LEUKORRHEA - A whitish sticky discharge from the vagina and uterine cavity.

LITHIC MATERIAL - Refers to the calculus or stoney build-up in the kidney or urinary bladder.

MACERATE - The softening of a solid by soaking. Used as a step in the extracting of plant medicines.

MALARIAL PERIODICITY - The regular recurrence of the intensified symptoms of malaria.

MARC - The residue or spent plant remains after maceration and perculation.

MASTITIS - Inflammation of the breast or mammary gland.

MEDICAMENT - A medicinal substance or agent.

MENORRHAGIA - Excessive uterine bleeding; the period of flow being greater than usual or normal.

METRITIS - Inflammation of the uterus.

METRORRHAGIA - Uterine bleeding of normal amounts, but occurring at completely irregular intervals.

MINIMS - Refers to a drop of liquid. Usually $\frac{1}{16}$th of a fluid dram.

MISSISSIPPIAN - A geologic time period in the Paleozoic era.

MUCUS (MUCOUS) - The free slime secreted by the glands of the mucous membranes.

MYOCARDITIS - Inflammation of the muscle tissue of the heart.

NARCOTIC - An agent that produces a deadening or numbing feeling or condition.

NEPHRITIS - Inflammation of the kidney.

NERVINE - An agent which relieves pain. (does not include morphine or the narcotics.)

NERVE TONIC - An agent which tones or strengthens the nerves.

NEUROTOXIC - A poison to the nerve cells or to the nervous system.

OPHTHALMIA - A severe inflammation of the eye or conjunctiva.

OVATE - A botanical description of leaf shape which is "egg-shaped".

PALEOZOIC - A broad expanse of time (designated as an Era), with smaller subdivisions of time called periods. *(Paleo* = Old + *Zoic* = Animal)

PALPITATION - An unduly rapid action of the heart which is felt by the individual.

PARTURIENT - Pertains to the birth process; or sometimes designates a woman in labor.

PARTURITION - The act of giving birth to a child.

PARTUS PREPARATUS - An agent which diminishes false labor pains and produces effectual uterine contractions.

180

PATHOGENIC - Generally refers to an agent which causes sickness or a morbid condition.

PECTORAL - Pertains to the breast or chest area.

PELVIC NEURALGIA - Pain in the lower part of the trunk or body torso.

PERENNIAL - Refers to a plant's life-cycle in which it grows year after year.

PERICARDITIS - Inflammation of the membrane which surrounds the heart.

PERISTALTIC ACTION - The wave-like action of the esophagus, stomach and intestine which moves alimentary products through the system.

PETIOLATE - Refers to a leaf petal with a stalk or stem.

PISTILLATE FLOWER - The term describes a female flower. An imperfect flower without male parts.

PLEURISY - Inflammation of the serous membrane which lines the lungs and thoracic cavity.

PNEUMONIA - Inflammation of the lungs caused by a bacteria in the genus *Pneumococcus.*

POULTICE - A soft, moist mass of material applied (usually hot) to the surface of the skin for the purpose of supplying heat and moisture to enhance the healing function of the body.

PRE-PARTURITION - Before the actual time of labor and fetal delivery.

PROSTATIC HYPERTROPHY - A morbid enlargement or over-growth of the prostrate gland.

PROSTATIC - Pertains to the prostrate gland.

PROTHROMBIC - Pertains to prothrombin, a glycoprotein factor in the blood which is necessary for coagulation (Clotting).

PSORIASIS - A scaling skin disease.

PULMONARY CATARRH - Inflammation of the mucous membranes of the lungs and its secretions.

PULVERIZING - The reduction of any substance to a powder or near powder form.

PUNGENT - Sharp or biting olfactory sensation. Somewhat acrid.

PURULENT - Containing pus; or associated with the formation of pus.

PYORRHEA - Purulent inflammation of the membrane which holds the tooth in its socket. (Periodontal membrane).

Q.I.D. - Latin abbreviation for *quater in die,* 4 times a day.

REFRIGERANT - A cooling remedy; an agent relieving fever or thirst.

RELAXANT - An agent that lessens tension, especially muscle tension.

RENAL ANTISEPTIC - An agent which destroys kidney type bacterial infections.

RENAL CATARRH - Inflammation of the kidney mucous membranes with a free discharge of inflammed mucous material.

RENAL CYSTIC - Pertains to the kidney and urinary bladder.

RENAL MUCOSA - The mucous secreting cells which line the kidney ducts, etc.

RENAL SEDATIVE - An agent which allays or calms the kidneys.

RHEUMATIC - Pertains to the inflammatory condition of the connective tissue structures and of the muscles and joints associated with the tissue.

RHIZOMES - These are underground horizontal stems.

RHUS POISONING - Poison by touching. Air or smoke contact with the volatile oils of poison oak, poison ivy, etc.

RUBEFACIENT - An agent that reddens the skin (hyperemia).

SCORBUTIC DISEASE - A Vitamin C related disease; scurvy.

SCROFULA - Tuberculosis of the lymphatic glands. Usually a disease of early life.

SCURVY - A Vitamin C deficiency disease.

SEDATIVE - A calming agent.

SEPTICEMIA - Presence in the blood of bacterial toxins or poisons.

STAMINATE FLOWER - Imperfect flower with the male structures (stamens) only.

STAPHLACOCCUS - A disease bacteria. They are characterized by their clumping formation.

STEEP - To soak in a liquid at a temperature under the boiling point.

STIMULANT - An agent or remedy that produces stimulation, especially of the muscle fibers through action of the nervous tissue.

STOMACHIC - An agent or medicine which promotes the functional activities of the stomach.

STONES - A mass of extremely hard material located in the kidney or associated organs.

STREP THROAT - A sore throat caused by the streptococci bacteria.

STROBILUS - A cone-like reproductive structure bearing spores.

STY - Inflammation of one or more sebaceous glands of he eyelids.

STYPTIC - An astringent or hemostatic remedy which arrests bInflammation of one or more sebaceous glands of the eyelids.

STYPTIC - An astringent or hemostatic remedy which arrests bleeding by means of its astringent quality.

SUPPURATION - The formation of pus; the act of becoming converted into pus.

TETANUS - An infectious disease caused by a bacterial toxin which causes sustained muscle contraction of the jaw muscle (Lock jaw).

THERAPEUTIC - The art of healing; or to render a cure.

T.I.D. - Latin for *ter in die;* take three times a day.

THYROID DYSFUNCTION - An impairment or disturbance in the functioning of the thyroid gland.

TONIC - A medicinal agent or preparation which restores normal tone to the tissue or organ.

TRAUMATIC - Pertains to a wound or injury.

URETHRITIS - An inflammation of the membranous canal which conveys urine from the bladder to the body's exterior.

UTERINE SUBINVOLUTION - Failure of the uterus to return to its normal size and condition after normal, functional enlargement.

VAGINITIS - Inflammation of the vagina.

VAGINAL MUCOSA - The mucous membrane lining of the vagina.

VASO-CONSTRICTOR - An agent or substance which causes the blood vessels to become smaller in diameter.

VISCOUS JUICE - A juice which has a sticky, thick appearance or property.

VULNERARY - An agent which is active in the healing of wounds.

WEEPING ECZEMA - Skin inflammation characterized by a watery discharge from the sore or lesion.

WHOOPING COUGH - An infectious disease characterized by mucous secretions of the respiratory tract, resulting in a whooping sound.

FROM THE SHEPHERD'S PURSE
INDEX

186

FROM THE SHEPHERD'S PURSE - PLANT LIST

COMMON NAME:	SCIENTIFIC NAME:	PLANT FAMILY:
1. Shepherd's Purse	Capsella bursa-pastoris	Cruciferae
2. Comfrey	Symphytum officinale	Boraginaceae
3. Mullein	Verbascum thapsus	Scrophulariaceae
4. Garlic	Allium sativum	Liliaceae
5. Red Clover	Trifolium pratense	Leguminosae
6. Spearmint	Mentha spicata	Labiatae
7. Peppermint	Mentha piperita	Labiatae
8. Catnip	Nepeta cataria	Labiatae
9. Horsemint	Monarda punctata	Labiatae
10. Pennyroyal	Hedeoma pulegioides	Labiatae
11. Plantain	Plantago major	Plantaginaceae
12. Rose Hips	Rosa woodsii	Rosaceae
13. Oregon Grape	Mahonia aquifolium	Berberidaceae
14. Shave Grass	Equisetum arvense	Equisetaceae
15. Juniper Berries	Juniperus communis	Cupressaceae
16. Life Root	Senecio aureus	Compositae
17. Tansey	Tanacetum vulgare	Compositae
18. Burdock	Arctium lappa	Compositae
19. Arnica	Arnica alpina	Compositae
20. Golden Seal	Hydrastis canadensis	Ranunculaceae
21. Lobelia	Lobelia inflata	Campanulaceae
22. Black Cohosh	Cimicifuga racemosa	Ranunculaceae
23. Raspberry	Rubus strigosis	Rosaceae
24. Squaw Vine	Mitchella repens	Rubiaceae
25. Scullcap	Scutellaria lateriflora	Labiatae
26. Yellow Dock	Rumex crispus	Polygonaceae
27. Bearberry	Arctostaphylos uva-ursi	Ericaceae
28. Gravel Root	Eupatorium purpureum	Compositae
29. Chickweed	Stellaria media	Caryophyllaceae
30. Camomile	Anthemis nobilis	Compositae
31. Iris	Iris versicolor	Iridaceae
32. Lady Slipper	Cypripedium pubescens	Orchidaceae
33. Couchgrass	Agropyron repens	Gramineae
34. Yarrow	Achillea millefolium	Compositae
35. Dandelion	Taraxacum officinale	Compositae
36. Flax	Linum lewisii	Linaceae
37. Elderberry	Sambucus nigra	Caprifoliaceae
38. Willow	Salix discolor	Salicaceae
39. Blue Cohosh	Caulophyllum thalictroides	Berberidaceae
40. Brigham Tea	Ephedra viridis	Ephedraceae
41. Aloe	Aloe vera	Liliaceae
42. Purple Coneflower	Echinaceae angustifolia	Compositae
43. Gumweed	Grindelia squarrosa	Compositae
44. Yellow Clover	Melilotus officinalis	Leguminosae
45. Bistort	Polygonum bistortoides	Polygonaceae
46. Cinquefoil	Potentilla fruticosa	Rosaceae
47. Chicory	Cichorium intybus	Compositae
48. Cayenne	Capsicum	Solanaceae